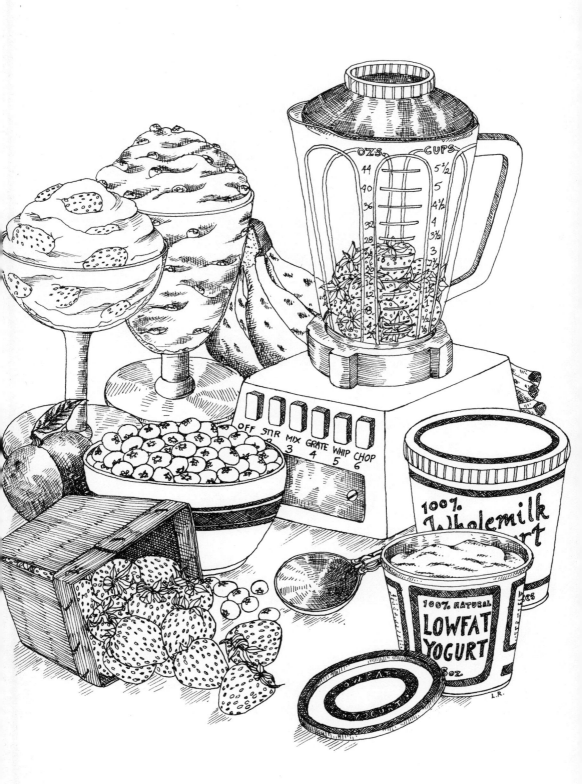

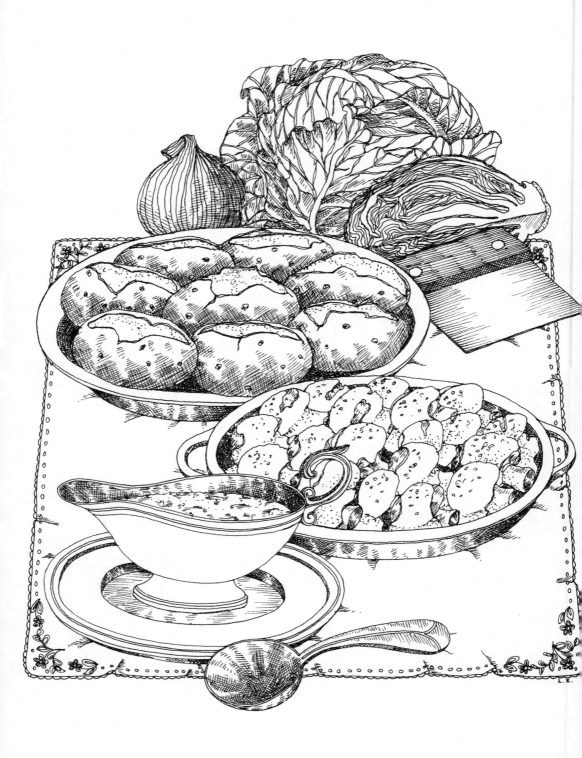

The American Diabetes Association
The American Dietetic Association
FAMILY COOKBOOK

Illustrated by Lauren Rosen

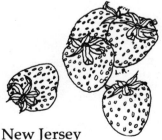

Prentice-Hall, Inc., Englewood Cliffs, New Jersey
Robert J. Brady Co., Bowie, Maryland

Book Designer: Joan Ann Jacobus
Art Director: Hal Siegel

The American Diabetes Association/
The American Dietetic Association Family Cookbook by The American Diabetes Association/
The American Dietetic Association
Copyright © 1980 by The American Diabetes Association/
The American Dietetic Association

Library of Congress Cataloging in Publication Data

American Diabetes Association.
    The American Diabetes Association, the American
Dietetic Association family cookbook.

    Bibliography: p.
    Includes index.
    1. Diabetes—Diet therapy—Recipes.   I. American
Dietetic Association.   II. Title.   III. Title: Family
cookbook.
RC662.A43   1980   641.5′6314   80-16722
ISBN 0-13-024901-7

Contents

Foreword

Proper nutrition is essential to good health. The basics of good nutrition apply to both individuals with diabetes and those without. This volume provides a resource of nutritious recipes for diabetics as well as for their families and the entire community. Everyone uses glucose (blood sugar) as fuel for energy. However, people with diabetes differ in that their bodies cannot store and use glucose as efficiently; in addition they make more glucose from other food stuffs than nondiabetic persons. To avoid high blood sugar, diabetics must pay stricter attention to what they eat, how much, and when. Also individuals with diabetes traditionally have avoided or limited foods high in sucrose (table sugar). Other than that, however, individuals with diabetes are encouraged to eat the same foods as everyone else. In fact, the distribution of carbohydrate, protein, and fat in the diets of people with diabetes should match that of nondiabetics. This book was written in response to many requests from diabetics who intuitively knew that their diets would be good for everyone and who wanted a cookbook that the whole family could use. In developing the book, The American Diabetes Association enlisted the help of dietitians all across the country. Special thanks, however, go to the Nutrition Committee of the Michigan Affiliate, whose time and effort made this book a reality. Other Affiliates and individual dietitians around the country contributed immeasurably to the manuscript. We believe this book is the definitive nutrition guide and cookbook for people who must control carbohydrates and calories, and particularly for families of diabetics. We're pleased we've been able to answer a long unmet need.

Ronald A. Arky, M.D.
President
The American Diabetes Association

The American Dietetic Association is pleased to collaborate with The American Diabetes Association in the preparation of this practical, highly informative cookbook and nutrition guide. We feel it is destined to become a classic of its kind. It is more than a cookbook: It is a guide to good eating and nutritional health applicable to healthy persons as well as those with diabetes. Students of nutrition and other health professionals will find succinct, useful information in the sections on normal nutrition, exercise, weight control, and meal planning. Dietitians and physicians will find a ready reference book that is useful for persons with diabetes as well as their families. The Association proudly presents this first edition of *The Family Cookbook* and acknowledges the efforts of the many persons who prepared the manuscript and reviewed the material for publication.

Esther Winterfeldt, Ph.D., R.D.
President
The American Dietetic Association

Introduction

This book is a wonderful treasury of delicious, nutritious, and economical recipes for use in planning meals of people who must control carbohydrates and calories, particularly those who have diabetes mellitus. Moreover, it is something greater than that. As you look at the more than 250 recipes, notice that the ingredients are ordinary foods—even sugar in measured amounts.

The recipes are designed to yield four to six servings. Exchange equivalents have been calculated for single servings for all recipes and are listed with the recipe. This information will help you adapt a given recipe to the Exchange or meal plan. The amount of protein, fat, carbohydrate, and calories for a single serving of each recipe is included along with its sodium and potassium contents.

This book also is a guide to sound nutrition. It explains what "good nutrition" means and why it's important. Take some time to become familiar with the introductory chapters. If you are just beginning to live with diabetes or with a calorie or carbohydrate limit, they will help you understand why eating wisely is a part of good health management; it facilitates good diabetic control and results in a general feeling of well-being. If, on the other hand, you have lived with diabetes or a carbohydrate/calorie limit for many years, they will offer ways to broaden the variety in your menus and help you cope with many diet-related situations of daily living.

The material incorporates the latest information about the role of nutrition in the management of diabetes, including carbohydrate and calorie control, as well as important nutritional information applicable to the whole family. The guidelines contained herein are approved by the individuals and committees listed below, and we extend our appreciation to them for their contributions.

Acknowledgements

The American Diabetes Association and The American Dietetic Association gratefully acknowledge the contributions made by:

Members of The American Dietetic Association.

Members of the American Diabetes Association Affiliates in Michigan, Connecticut (in conjunction with the Connecticut Dietetic Association), Cincinnati, Southern California, Tennessee (Knox Area Chapter), Georgia, North Texas, and Arizona.

A special thanks is extended to the staff and students in the Dietetics Program at Madonna College in Michigan for their assistance with laboratory recipe testing, and to the many families who home-tested the recipes.

Affiliate Associations of the American Diabetes Association

American Diabetes Association
Alabama Affiliate, Inc.
Huntsville, Alabama

American Diabetes Association
Alaska Affiliate, Inc.
Anchorage, Alaska

American Diabetes Association
Arizona Affiliate, Inc.
Phoenix, Arizona

American Diabetes Association
Arkansas Affiliate, Inc.
Little Rock, Arkansas

American Diabetes Association
Southern California Affiliate, Inc.
Los Angeles, California

American Diabetes Association
Northern California Affiliate, Inc.
San Francisco, California

American Diabetes Association
Colorado Affiliate, Inc.
Denver, Colorado

American Diabetes Association
Connecticut Affiliate, Inc.
West Hartford, Connecticut

American Diabetes Association
Delaware Affiliate, Inc.
Wilmington, Delaware

American Diabetes Association
Washington, D.C. Area
    Affiliate, Inc.
Silver Spring, Maryland

American Diabetes Association
Florida Affiliate, Inc.
Orlando, Florida

American Diabetes Association
Georgia Affiliate, Inc.
Atlanta, Georgia

American Diabetes Association
Hawaii Affiliate, Inc.
Honolulu, Hawaii

American Diabetes Association
Idaho Affiliate, Inc.
Boise, Idaho

American Diabetes Association
Northern Illinois Affiliate, Inc.
Chicago, Illinois

American Diabetes Association
Minnesota Affiliate, Inc.
Minneapolis, Minnesota

American Diabetes Association
Downstate Illinois Affiliate, Inc.
Decatur, Illinois

American Diabetes Association
Mississippi Affiliate, Inc.
Jackson, Mississippi

American Diabetes Association
Indiana Affiliate, Inc.
Indianapolis, Indiana

American Diabetes Association
Missouri Regional Affiliate, Inc.
Columbia, Missouri

American Diabetes Association
Iowa Affiliate, Inc.
Cedar Rapids, Iowa

American Diabetes Association
Heart of America Affiliate, Inc.
Kansas City, Missouri

American Diabetes Association
Kansas Affiliate, Inc.
Wichita, Kansas

American Diabetes Association
Greater St. Louis Affiliate, Inc.
St. Louis, Missouri

American Diabetes Association
Kentucky Affiliate, Inc.
Lexington, Kentucky

American Diabetes Association
Montana Affiliate, Inc.
Great Falls, Montana

American Diabetes Association
Louisiana Affiliate, Inc.
Baton Rouge, Louisiana

American Diabetes Association
Nebraska Affiliate, Inc.
Omaha, Nebraska

American Diabetes Association
Maryland Affiliate, Inc.
Baltimore, Maryland

American Diabetes Association
Nevada Affiliate, Inc.
Las Vegas, Nevada

American Diabetes Association
New England Affiliate, Inc.
Newton Upper Falls, Mass.

American Diabetes Association
New Hampshire Affiliate, Inc.
Concord, New Hampshire

American Diabetes Association
Michigan Affiliate, Inc.
Detroit, Michigan

American Diabetes Association
New Jersey Affiliate, Inc.
Hackensack, New Jersey

American Diabetes Association
New Mexico Affiliate, Inc.
Albuquerque, New Mexico

American Diabetes Association
Western New York Affiliate, Inc.
Buffalo, New York

American Diabetes Association
New York Diabetes Affiliate, Inc.
New York, New York

American Diabetes Association
Rochester Regional Affiliate, Inc.
Rochester, New York

American Diabetes Association
Upstate New York Chapter, Inc.
Syracuse, New York

American Diabetes Association
Central New York Chapter, Inc.
Utica, New York

American Diabetes Association
North Carolina Affiliate, Inc.
Charlotte, North Carolina

American Diabetes Association
North Dakota Affiliate, Inc.
Grand Forks, North Dakota

American Diabetes Association
Akron Area Affiliate, Inc.
Akron, Ohio

American Diabetes Association
Greater Ohio Affiliate, Inc.
Arlington, Ohio

American Diabetes Association
Cincinnati Affiliate, Inc.
Cincinnati, Ohio

American Diabetes Association
Dayton Area Affiliate, Inc.
Dayton, Ohio

American Diabetes Association
Mahoning Valley Chapter, Inc.
Youngstown, Ohio

American Diabetes Association
Southeastern Ohio Chapter, Inc.
Zanesville, Ohio

American Diabetes Association
Western Oklahoma Chapter, Inc.
Oklahoma City, Oklahoma

American Diabetes Association
Eastern Oklahoma Chapter, Inc.
Tulsa, Oklahoma

American Diabetes Association
Oregon Affiliate, Inc.
Portland, Oregon

American Diabetes Association
Pennsylvania Affiliate, Inc.
Allentown, Pennsylvania

American Diabetes Association
Greater Philadelphia Affiliate, Inc.
Philadelphia, Pennsylvania

American Diabetes Association
Western Penna. Affiliate, Inc.
Pittsburgh, Pennsylvania

American Diabetes Association
Rhode Island Affiliate, Inc.
Providence, Rhode Island

American Diabetes Association
South Carolina Affiliate, Inc.
Greenville, South Carolina

American Diabetes Association
South Dakota Affiliate, Inc.
Sioux Falls, South Dakota

American Diabetes Association
Memphis Mid-South
    Affiliate, Inc.
Memphis, Tennessee

American Diabetes Association
Greater Tennessee Affiliate, Inc.
Nashville, Tennessee

American Diabetes Association
South Texas Affiliate, Inc.
Austin, Texas

American Diabetes Association
North Texas Affiliate, Inc.
Dallas, Texas

American Diabetes Association
Utah Affiliate, Inc.
Salt Lake City, Utah

American Diabetes Association
Vermont Affiliate, Inc.
Burlington, Vermont

American Diabetes Association
Virginia Affiliate, Inc.
Virginia Beach, Virginia

American Diabetes Association
Washington Affiliate, Inc.
Seattle, Washington

American Diabetes Association
West Virginia Affiliate, Inc.
Charleston, West Virginia

American Diabetes Association
Wisconsin Affiliate, Inc.
Milwaukee, Wisconsin

American Diabetes Association
Wyoming Affiliate, Inc.
Cheyenne, Wyoming

The American Dietetic Association has state Associations in each state, and district Associations in many areas. Your local American Diabetes Association Affiliate can provide you the current address of The Dietetic Association nearest you.

1 □ THE BASICS OF GOOD NUTRITION

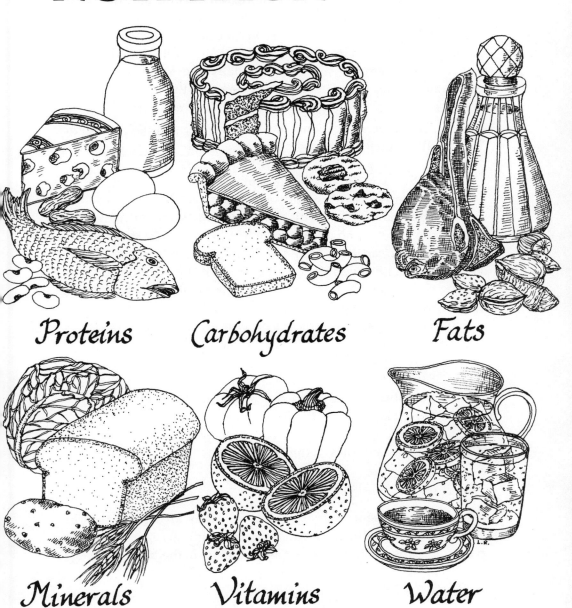

Proteins   Carbohydrates   Fats

Minerals   Vitamins   Water

Good eating is not only fun, it is also necessary for good nutrition. Eating a sufficient variety of wholesome foods supplies the body with energy in the form of calories and approximately fifty different known nutrients which are the building blocks of thousands of substances necessary for healthful living. If the body could manufacture those nutrients on its own, we wouldn't have to eat at all! But of course it must obtain them from food. For all healthy individuals the nutrient requirements are fundamentally the same, varying primarily in *amounts* during the various stages of the life cycle. Table 1 shows a family plan for good nutrition at different ages.

The different nutrients have different functions, but together they do three major jobs in the body:

1. Provide energy, measured in calories.
2. Build, maintain, repair, and replace body tissues.
3. Help to regulate body processes.

The individual with diabetes needs the same nutrients as the rest of the family, and today there are many foods from which a nutritious diet can be selected. All of it can be purchased in the grocery store; no special food is required for the diabetic person. In buying food, just remember that no single food is nutritionally perfect. A good variety is needed for good nutrition.

The six major groups of nutrients are:

Proteins
Carbohydrates
Fats
Vitamins
Minerals
Water

Each plays specific roles in the body.

PROTEIN

Proteins are present in every living cell; they are essential to life. The body uses proteins for building, maintaining, repairing, and replacing tissues. Proteins also act as regulators in the body, helping to

TABLE 1 A FAMILY PLAN FOR GOOD NUTRITION

Food Classes	Amount Each Day			Major Nutrients Provided
	Adult	Teen	Child	
Milk and milk products	2 cups	4 cups	2–3 cups	Protein, fat, calcium, riboflavin, vitamins A, D
Meat, fish, poultry, eggs, dried beans	4–6 ounces	4–6 ounces	2–4 ounces	Protein, fat, niacin, iron, thiamine, and other vitamins and minerals
Deep green and yellow vegetables and fruits includes: broccoli, carrots, pumpkin, winter squash, sweet potatoes, spinach, turnip greens, and other green leafy vegetables. Also apricots, cantaloupe, and peaches	1 serving at least every other day			Vitamin A, other vitamins, and fiber
Citrus fruits includes: tomatoes, oranges, grapefruit, lemons, lime	1 serving every day			Vitamin C, other vitamins, and fiber
Potatoes and other fruits and vegetables	2 servings every day			Vitamins, minerals, and fiber
Whole grains or enriched breads, cereals, pasta	At least 4 servings			Carbohydrates, thiamine, niacin, riboflavin, iron, and fiber
Other foods includes: margarine, butter, other fats, simple desserts (gelatin, pudding, plain cakes, and cookies)	Amount depends on daily caloric needs			Fat and fat soluble vitamins, calories to round out the day's needs

keep the body's chemistry balanced. They are a part of such substances as hormones (including insulin) and antibodies.

The building blocks of proteins are the twenty-two amino acids. Nine of these cannot be manufactured by the body in sufficient amounts and must be provided by foods. These are called the *essential amino acids* (EAA).

Amino acids are found in animal and plant sources. Animal sources (meat, fish, poultry, eggs, and cheese) supply "complete" proteins; that is, they contain the nine essential amino acids in amounts needed by the body. Plant sources (dried peas, beans, nuts, seeds, grains, and cereals) are short in one or more essential amino acids. You can meet your needs for amino acids by combining different plant sources so the essential amino acids short in one plant are supplied by a second plant source. Plant protein may also be combined with animal protein to enhance its value to the body. Unlike most animal proteins, plant proteins also contain carbohydrate.

Examples of plant combinations which provide complete protein are:

Corn bread and garbanzo beans

Split pea and barley soup

Whole wheat bread and peanut butter

Lentils and rice

Corn and lima beans

The body's highest priority is for energy. If *too few* carbohydrate and fat calories are eaten to supply the energy needs, protein will be used for energy rather than for the functions listed above. When *excess* protein calories are eaten, they are broken down by the body and stored as fat.

CARBOHYDRATES

Carbohydrate-rich foods are the cheapest and the most efficient source of energy for the body. On the basis of their complexity, carbohydrates are subdivided into three groups: monosaccharides, disaccharides, and polysaccharides. The term *sugar* usually is applied to monosaccharides and disaccharides, and the term *complex carbohydrates* usually refers to polysaccharides (such as starch).

Examples of foods rich in sugar (monosaccharides and disaccharides):

Honey

Syrup

Candy

Corn syrup

Table sugar

Jam, jelly, marmalade

Cakes, pies, cookies, molasses

Sweetened carbonated beverages

Gelatine dessert

Examples of foods rich in complex carbohydrates (polysaccharides):

Bread

Cereal

Vegetables

Pasta

Rice

Fruit and milk, although containing monosaccharides and disaccharides, are not classified with other foods listed in these categories but are treated separately.

Some carbohydrate-rich foods contain a constituent called *fiber,* which appears to have certain health benefits. Whole-grain breads and cereals (wheat, rye, oats, barley), vegetables, and fruits (especially skins and edible seeds)—major dietary sources of fiber—help prevent constipation. Fiber adds bulk to the diet and gives a feeling of fullness, a welcome plus for people who want to control their weight and thus must cut down on the amount of food they eat.

FATS

Some fat is essential in the diet and it is found in both animal and plant food. Foods rich in fat from plant sources include margarine, oil (vegetable, salad, cooking), salad dressing, and nuts. Some products that contain animal fats are meats, fish, poultry, eggs, butter, milk, and cheese. In general, fish, chicken, and turkey are lower in fat than the red meats (pork, beef, and lamb). Milk and cheese are available with a reduced fat content; examples include fortified skim and low fat milk, and cheese made from skim or partially skim milk (such as cottage, Swiss, hoop, and mozzarella cheese).

Foods rich in fats are the most concentrated source of calories. Weight for weight, fats supply more than twice as much energy as carbohydrates and protein. Dietary fats supply an essential fatty acid that the body cannot make. The fat in many foods is a carrier of fat soluble vitamins. Foods high in fat often make people feel satisfied longer because digestion takes longer.

Cholesterol, saturated fats, and polyunsaturated fats are the focus of much interest today, because they may play a role in heart and blood vessel disease such as atherosclerosis, a disease in which a thickening and narrowing of the arteries (major blood vessels) occurs. These mushy deposits of fat, cholesterol, and other materials in the inner layer of the arterial wall interfere with the normal blood flow and nourishment of tissues.

Cholesterol is manufactured in the human body and it is also obtained from foods of animal origin. Egg yolks and organ meats (liver, kidney, brains, and sweetbreads) are particularly high in cholesterol. All fish and shellfish are low in cholesterol except shrimp and sardines. Foods of plant origin have no cholesterol.

Saturated animal fats are found in beef, lamb, pork, ham, butter, cream, whole milk, and whole-milk cheeses. Saturated vegetable fats are found in hydrogenated shortenings, palm oil, cocoa butter, and coconut oil. Most of these fats harden at room temperature. High consumption of saturated fats may contribute to heart and blood vessel disease because it tends to raise the level of cholesterol in the blood, and excessive cholesterol in the circulation has been implicated in these diseases.

Polyunsaturated fats—usually liquid oils of vegetable origin, such as corn, cottonseed, sunflower, and safflower oil—tend to lower the level of cholesterol in the blood.

Monounsaturated oils, such as olive oil and peanut oil, neither raise nor lower serum cholesterol.

VITAMINS

Vitamins are necessary for growth, cell reproduction, normal functioning of the gastrointestinal tract, mental alertness, and resistance to infection, just to mention a few of their functions. The known vitamins include the following:

WATER-SOLUBLE VITAMINS
Vitamin C (ascorbic acid), Thiamine (B_1), Ribloflavin (B_2), Niacin (B_3), Pyridoxine, Pantothenic Acid, Biotin, Vitamin B_{12}, Folacin, Choline.

FAT-SOLUBLE VITAMINS
Vitamin A, Vitamin D, Vitamin E, Vitamin K.
Functions of several of these vitamins are defined and presented in Table 2 along with some foods that provide them. Necessary vitamins may be obtained by eating a variety of foods. Excess amounts of Vitamins A and D can be harmful, so supplements should be taken only when prescribed by a physician.

Water-soluble vitamins taken in amounts greater than the body's need are excreted in the urine. Supplements in addition to a good diet are probably a waste of money.

MINERALS

Some of the varied functions of minerals include aiding normal functioning of nerves and muscles, regulating many body processes, and aiding the formation of bones and contributing to their strength. They are classified as *microminerals* or *macrominerals*. Microminerals (often referred to as *trace minerals*) are necessary to the body in very small amounts. Examples of such minerals are iron, zinc, and fluorine. Examples of macrominerals are calcium, magnesium, phosphorus, sodium, and potassium. Macrominerals are those occurring in appreciable amounts in the body, accounting for most of the body content of minerals.

Adequate minerals may be obtained from carefully selected food sources. Like some vitamins, excessive amounts of certain minerals can be harmful. So mineral supplements should be taken only when prescribed by a physician. Functions and food sources of several minerals are shown in Table 2.

TABLE 2 VITAMINS, MINERALS, AND YOU

WHY YOU NEED THEM	FOODS THAT SUPPLY THEM
VITAMIN C (Ascorbic Acid): Helps hold body cells together and strengthens walls of blood cells. Helps in wound healing. Helps body to build bones and teeth. Helps in absorption and use of iron.	Cantaloupe, grapefruit, oranges, strawberries, broccoli, cabbage, tomatoes, green leafy vegetables, and fresh potatoes.
THIAMINE (B_1): Helps body cells obtain energy from food. Helps keep nerves in healthy condition. Promotes good appetite and digestion.	Whole-grain and enriched breads, cereals, potatoes, organ meats, pork, other meats, poultry and fish, nuts, milk, green vegetables, dried peas, and beans.
RIBOFLAVIN (B_2): Helps cells use oxygen to release energy from food. Helps keep eyes healthy. Helps keep skin around mouth and nose healthy.	Milk, liver, kidney, heart, lean meat, eggs, and green leafy greens, enriched and whole-grain breads and cereals.
NIACIN (B_3): Helps the cells of the body use oxygen to produce energy. Maintains health of skin, tongue, digestive tract, and nervous system.	Liver, poultry, fish, lean meat, peanuts and peanut butter, beans and peas, and whole-grain and enriched breads and cereals.

WHY YOU NEED THEM	FOODS THAT SUPPLY THEM
VITAMIN B_{12}: Helps with normal functioning of all body cells. Necessary for formation of red blood cells.	Liver, other organ meats, fish, meat, eggs, shellfish, milk, cottage cheese, and other milk products, except butter.
VITAMIN A: Helps keep eyes healthy and able to adjust to dim light. Keeps skin healthy. Helps keep lining of mouth, nose, throat, and digestive tract healthy and resistant to infection. Promotes growth.	Liver, dark green and deep yellow vegetables such as broccoli, collards, and other dark green leafy vegetables, carrots, pumpkin, sweet potatoes, winter squash, tomatoes, green pepper, apricots, cantaloupe, strawberries, papaya, watermelon, butter, and fortified margarine.
VITAMIN D: Promotes growth and lays down minerals for bones and teeth.	Egg yolk, butter, fortified margarine, fortified milk, fatty fish, and liver. Vitamin D is produced in the skin with the stimulus of sunlight.
VITAMIN E: Helps other vitamins and unsaturated fatty acids perform their special functions in the body. Helps protect red blood cells from oxidation.	Fats and polyunsaturated oils of vegetable products, safflower oil. Meats and green vegetables contain small amounts. Whole-grain cereals and peanuts.
IRON: Combines with protein to make hemoglobin, the red substance of blood which carries oxygen from the lungs to muscles, brain, and other parts of the body. Helps cells use oxygen. Prevents anemia.	Liver, kidney, heart, oysters, lean meat, egg yolk, dried beans, dried peas, dark green leafy vegetables, dried fruit, whole-grain and enriched bread and cereals, and prune juice.
CALCIUM: Builds bones and teeth. Helps blood to clot. Helps nerves, muscles, and heart to function properly.	Milk: fortified skim, low-fat, whole, buttermilk, yogurt; cheeses made from skim or partially skim milk (mozzarella), whole-milk cheese (Cheddar); leafy vegetables such as collards, dandelion, kale, mustard, and turnip greens.

TABLE 2 VITAMINS, MINERALS, AND YOU (continued)

WHY YOU NEED THEM	FOODS THAT SUPPLY THEM
MAGNESIUM: Activates various enzymes. Aids in energy production and utilization, contraction of nerves and muscles, and building tissue.	Bananas, whole-grain cereals, dried beans, milk, most dark green vegetables, meat, nuts, peanuts and peanut butter.
ZINC: Is a constituent of the hormone insulin. Activates various enzymes. Aids in growth, wound healing and prevention of anemia, taste acuity.	Whole grains, dried beans and peas, nuts, shellfish (particularly oysters), meat, cheese, and cocoa.
SODIUM: Is a key element in regulation of body water and of acid-base balance in the body	Some present in all natural foods; broth, gelatin dessert, table salt, baking soda, and most processed foods.
POTASSIUM: Is a component of lean body tissue. Contributes to growth and muscle strength. Helps regulate body water and acid-base balance. Helps maintain neuro-muscular function.	Meats, milk, fruits (especially citrus fruits), bananas, dried dates, cantaloupe, apricots, tomato juice, potatoes, and dark green leafy vegetables.

The presence or absence of vitamins and minerals in the diet can mean the difference between normal and abnormal functioning of the body. Because sodium and potassium are minerals found in almost all foods, it is important to examine them more closely.

SODIUM

Most foods have some naturally occurring sodium as well as that added in processing. But the major source of dietary sodium is sodium chloride (table salt). Sodium chloride, or salt, is frequently eaten in excess. Under unusual conditions, if the kidneys (which rid the body of wastes) cannot get rid of the excess sodium, the sodium may make the body cells retain fluid. Fluid retention, in turn, may aggravate high blood pressure and other medical problems.

If a doctor suggests sodium restriction, a diet counselor can help you avoid foods that should not be used and can help you switch seasonings creatively. If you are afraid that omitting salt will make the foods you serve taste flat or bland, don't despair. Herbs and spices open a whole new world of flavor and aroma. To enhance a low-salt or salt-free dish, use herbs and spices in combination or alone. Experiment; be creative. But remember it is easier to add more than to take some out if you've added too much. A simple rule of thumb is to add a small amount at a time and taste.

USES OF SPICES AND HERBS*

Spice	Uses
Allspice	Pot roast, fish, eggs, pickles, sweet potatoes, squash, fruit
Anise seed	Cookies, cakes, breads, candy, cheese, beverages, pickles, beef stew, stewed fruits, fish
Basil	Tomatoes, noodles, rice, beef stew, pork, meat loaf, duck, fish, veal, green or vegetable salad, eggplant, potatoes, carrots, spinach, peas, eggs, cheese, jelly
Bay leaf	Soups, chowders, pickles, fish, pot roast, variety meats, stews, marinades
Caraway seed	Green beans, beets, cabbage, carrots, cauliflower, potatoes, sauerkraut, turnips, zucchini, goose, lamb, pork, spareribs, beef or lamb stew, marinades for meats, cake, cookies, rice, rye bread
Cardamom	Baked goods, pickles, grape jelly, puddings, sweet potatoes, squash, fruit soups
Cayenne pepper	Meat dishes, spaghetti, pizza, chicken, fish, eggs, cheese, vegetables, pickles
Celery seed	Potato salad, fruit salad, tomatoes, vegetables, stuffings, pickles, breads, rolls, egg dishes, meat loaf, stews, soups.

*Adapted from the United States Department of Agriculture Research Service, Consumer and Food Economics Institute.

USES OF SPICES AND HERBS (continued)

Spice	Uses
Chili powder	Tomato or barbecue sauces, dips, egg dishes, stews, meat loaf, chicken, marinades for meats, cheese, bean casseroles, corn, eggplant
Cinnamon	Beverages, bakery products, fruits, pickles, pork, ham, lamb or beef stews, roast lamb, chicken
Cloves	Fruits, pickles, baked goods, fish, stuffings, meat sauces, pot roast, marinades for meats, green beans, Harvard beets, carrots, sweet potatoes, tomatoes; used whole to stud ham, fruit, glazed pork, beef
Curry powder	Curried beef, chicken, fish, lamb, meatballs, pork, veal, eggs, dried beans, fruit, dips, breads, marinades for meats
Dill seed	Pickles, pickled beets, salads, sauerkraut, green beans, egg dishes, stews, fish, chicken, breads
Fennel seed	Egg dishes, fish, stews, marinades for meats, vegetables, cheese, baked or stewed apples, pickles, sauerkraut, breads, cakes, cookies
Garlic	Tomato dishes, soups, dips, sauces, salads, salad dressings, dill pickles, meat, poultry, fish, stews, marinades, bread
Ginger	Pickles, conserves, baked or stewed fruits, vegetables, baked products, beef, lamb, pork, veal, poultry, fish, beverages, soups, Oriental dishes
Mace	Baked products, fruits, meat loaf, fish, poultry, chowder, vegetables, jellies, pickles, breads
Marjoram	Lamb, pork, beef, veal, chicken, fish, tomato dishes, carrots, cauliflower, peas, spinach, squash, mushrooms, broccoli, pizza, spaghetti, egg dishes, breads, soups

Spice	Uses
Mint	Punches, tea, sauces for desserts, sauces for lamb, mint jelly, sherbet, vegetables, lamb stew, lamb roast
Mustard (dry)	Egg and cheese dishes, salad dressings, meat, poultry, vegetables
Mustard seed	Cucumber pickles, corned beef, coleslaw, potato salad, boiled cabbage, sauerkraut
Nutmeg	Hot beverages, puddings, baked products, fruits, chicken, seafood, eggs, vegetables, pickles, conserves
Onion powder	Dips, soups, stews, all meats, fish, poultry, salads, vegetables, stuffing, cheese dishes, egg dishes, breads, rice dishes
Oregano	Tomatoes, pasta sauces, pizza, chili con carne, barbecue sauce, vegetable soup, egg and cheese dishes, onions, stuffings, pork, lamb, chicken, fish
Parsley	Soups, coleslaw, breads, tomato and meat sauces, stuffings, broiled or fried fish, meats, poultry
Pepper: Black	Meats, poultry, fish, eggs, vegetables, pickles
Cayenne	Meats, soups, cheese dishes, sauces, pickles, poultry, vegetables, spaghetti sauce, curried dishes, dips, tamale pie, barbecued beef and pork
White	White or light meats, vegetables, white sauces and mashed potatoes
Poppy seed	Pie crust, scrambled eggs, fruit compotes, cheese sticks, fruit salad dressings, cookies, cakes, breads, noodles. Sprinkle over top of fruit salads, vegetables, breads, cookies, and cakes.

USES OF SPICES AND HERBS (continued)

Spice	Uses
Poultry seasoning	Stuffings, poultry, veal, meat loaf, chicken soup
Rosemary	Lamb, poultry, veal, beef, pork, fish, soups, stews, marinades, potatoes, cauliflower, spinach, mushrooms, turnips, fruits, breads
Saffron	Baked goods, chicken, seafood, rice, curries
Sage	Stuffings for poultry, fish, and other meats, sauces, soups, chowders, poultry, fish, beef, pork, veal, marinades, lima beans, onions, eggplant, tomatoes, cheese, potatoes
Sesame seed	Sprinkle canapes, breads, cookies, casseroles, salads, noodles, soups, vegetables. Add to pie crust, pie fillings, cakes, cookies, dips, stuffings.
Tarragon	Sour cream sauces, casseroles, marinades, pot roasts, veal, lamb, poultry, fish, egg dishes
Thyme	Meat, poultry, fish, vegetables
Turmeric	Cakes, breads, curried meats, fish, poultry, egg dishes, rice dishes, pickles
Vanilla	Baked goods, beverages, puddings

These foods are very high to moderately high in sodium:

CONDIMENTS: table salt, sea salt, seasoning salts, meat tenderizers, monosodium glutamate, soy sauce, steak sauce, Worcestershire sauce, pickles, olives, prepared mustard, catsup, barbecue sauce, chili sauce, relishes, garlic salt, onion salt, celery salt, and prepared horseradish.

SNACK FOODS: potato chips, pretzels, salted or unsalted crackers, salted nuts, corn chips, cheese curls, taco chips and pork rinds, party spreads and dips.

MEAT AND MEAT SUBSTITUTES: bologna or other luncheon meat, Canadian bacon, canned meat (corned beef, luncheon meat), canned fish (tuna, salmon), dried or chipped meat, ham, hot dogs, sausage, cheese (natural and processed), creamed cottage cheese, low-fat cottage cheese, sardines, herring, salted and dried codfish, anchovies, caviar, koshered meats, peanut butter, canned or commercially frozen mixed dishes, and most processed foods.

MISCELLANEOUS FOODS: sauerkraut, canned tomato juice, broth, bouillon or bouillon cubes, soup (canned, dried, or frozen), tomato sauce, tartar sauce, bacon and bacon fat, cheese dips, party spreads and dips, salt pork, gravy (canned or dried), monosodium glutamate, baking soda, and baking powder.

Many of the above foods are available in a low-sodium form at supermarkets.

POTASSIUM

Potassium is common in foods, so meeting daily needs is easy. However, certain diuretic medications, which are taken by some people who have high blood pressure, tend to draw potassium, sodium, and fluid out of the body and thus cause a drop in the body's normal potassium level. Also, vomiting and diarrhea cause the body to lose potassium.

If a doctor suggests the use of more potassium-rich foods, choose from the following list of fruits and vegetables. (Milk, selected meats and poultry also provide potassium.) Remember to use only the amounts of food specified in the meal plan. Raw fruits and vegetables have more potassium than cooked.

YOUR *BEST* SOURCES OF POTASSIUM ARE:

Fruits

Apricots	Dried fruit:	Nectarine
Avocado	Apricots, Dates	Papaya
Banana	Prunes, Raisins	Prune juice
	Melon	Rhubarb

Vegetables

Asparagus	Celery	Potato cooked in skin
Beets	Greens	Pumpkin
Broccoli	Lentils	Tomato; raw, juice,*
Brussels Sprouts	Lima beans	cooked, canned*
Carrots	Pepper, green	Winter squash
Cauliflower		

GOOD SOURCES OF POTASSIUM ARE:

Fruits

Apple, raw	Fruit cocktail	Pear
Berries	Grapefruit	Pineapple
Cherries	Orange	Plum
Fig	Peach	Tangerine

Juices

Apple	Grapefruit	Orange
Apricot	Lemon	Pineapple
Grape	Lime	

Vegetables

Corn	Lettuce	Summer squash
Cucumber	Mushrooms	Turnip
Green peas		Wax beans

*Not usually included on a sodium-restricted diet.

WATER

The last nutrient is water. The body's need for water is second only to that for oxygen. One may live for weeks without food, but only for a few days without water. The body gets water from (1) water you drink, (2) beverages such as coffee, tea, carbonated drinks, (3) liquid foods such as fruit juice, milk, and soups, (4) water in foods (even those which appear dry), and (5) water released when carbohydrates, proteins, and fats are metabolized in the body.

A WORD ABOUT FOOD ENERGY

Everyone needs energy for body work such as "basal metabolism," breathing, heartbeat, kidney function, and so on, as well as for physical activity. Children also need energy for growth. This is provided by food and expressed in terms of kilocalories or Calories.* The number of calories a food provides depends on the number of grams of carbohydrate, protein, and fat the food contains. Each gram of carbohydrate provides 4 calories; each gram of protein also provides 4 calories; and each gram of fat supplies 9 calories. See the examples below:

NUTRIENTS				FOODS		
	Bread (1 slice)			Corned Beef (3 ounces)		
	Grams	Calories per gram	Total calories	Grams	Calories per gram	Total calories
Carbohydrate	15	× 4 =	60	0	× 4 =	0
Protein	2	× 4 =	8	21	× 4 =	84
Fat	0	× 9 =	0	24	× 9 =	216
Total calories			68			300

*Calorie with a small c is commonly used and has been used in this book. It is important to remember, however, that such designation refers to kilocalorie, a unit 1,000 times as large as the small calorie used in the science of chemistry and physics.

Alcohol is also a source of energy for the body and is covered in Chapter 11. Vitamins and minerals and water do not supply energy; they have no calories.

When you get more calories than you need, whether in the form of fat, carbohydrate, protein, or alcohol, this excess energy is converted into body fat and stored in various parts of the body.

2 □ FOOD AND DIABETES

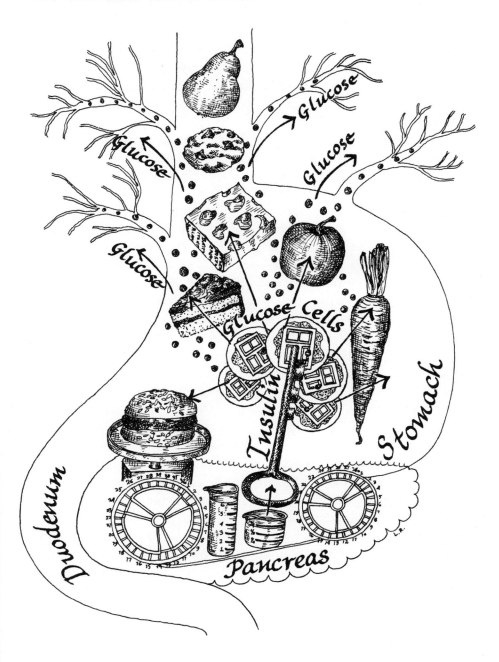

The basic nutrient and energy needs of all people are the same whether or not they have diabetes. However, individuals with diabetes must pay more attention to food since control of diet is a cornerstone of diabetic management. The foods for those with diabetes, in most instances, are much the same food as everyone else eats. However, because both exercise and medication for diabetes act to lower blood sugar, and because food raises blood sugar, the food has to be carefully selected and eaten at appropriate times to balance its effect.

When the body breaks down food in order to absorb it during digestion, the foods are converted to their simplest form for use by the body. Glucose is one of the end products of digestion. (Glucose is also the form in which sugar is present in the blood.) It serves as an energy source for the many different kinds of cells in the body. But for glucose to enter most cells, it needs the hormone insulin to let it in. *Insulin is the "key" that opens the cell "door."* Insulin is also necessary for the maintenance of the enzymic machinery required for the utilization of glucose inside the cell.

Normally, when glucose levels in the blood rise after eating, the pancreas releases insulin. This enables glucose to move from the bloodstream into the cell. However, when insulin is not available or doesn't work well, the glucose stays in the bloodstream and rises higher and higher (*hyperglycemia*, from *hyper* meaning high, *gly* meaning sugar, *emia* meaning blood) and eventually spills over into the urine (*glycosuria*, from *glycos* meaning sugar, *uria* meaning urine).

For one major class of diabetes, insulin-dependent diabetes, not enough insulin is produced to adequately move the glucose into the cells. In fact, often no insulin is produced at all. Therefore, these people must inject insulin one or more times a day. Therefore insulin is always in the bloodstream instead of being released in response to food. As a result, those who have diabetes and need insulin have to eat controlled amounts of food more frequently. A well-planned diet makes it possible to use insulin therapy more effectively and safely.

The other major class of diabetes is the non-insulin dependent, obese group. These individuals usually produce insulin, but the obesity interferes with the insulin's ability to work. A major goal of dietary treatment for this kind of diabetes is weight reduction. With loss of excess weight, nearly all in this group produce enough insulin to keep blood sugar levels normal.

DIETARY CONSTITUENTS

The calorie content of the diabetic meal plan should be enough to meet energy needs and at the same time keep weight within a normal range.

Most of the carbohydrate in a "diabetic meal" should come from foods that contain complex carbohydrates (polysaccharides), such as starchy foods. The amount of glucose and glucose containing disaccharides (sucrose, lactose) are restricted. In the "diabetic diet" 50 to 60 percent of calories are usually derived from carbohydrate, about the same amount suggested for the typical U.S. diet. The "diabetic diet" includes foods with complex carbohydrates (which have other nutrients) in preference to sugars (which have few other nutrients).

Individuals with diabetes are prone to develop premature cardiovascular disease. Although it is not certain that restriction of dietary saturated fat and cholesterol, and some use of polyunsaturated fats, will slow the progression of atherosclerosis, it is a reasonable expectation. Many with diabetes are advised to eat *less fat* and use foods with polyunsaturated fat in place of *some* foods with saturated fat. Saturated and polyunsaturated fats have the same number of calories, weight for weight. The Food Exchange Lists in the next chapter identify the various sources of fat.

The protein content of the diabetic meal plan should be adequate to meet growth and maintenance needs. Protein foods from plant sources and lean meats are low in fat content and will keep saturated fat intake low.

Vitamins and minerals are available in each meal plan to

meet ordinary needs: whole-grain breads, cereals, vegetables, fruits, dairy foods, meat, poultry, and fish are the major dietary sources of these nutrients.

SWEETENERS

Of special interest to anyone who must restrict carbohydrates and calories are saccharin and fructose.

Saccharin is a noncaloric sweetener. It is available straight and is used as an ingredient in many foods to reduce the sugar/calorie content. Its use by children and pregnant women should be discussed with the attending physician. A limited number of recipes using artificial sweetener have been included in this collection.

Fructose is a caloric sweetener. The body handles it and several sugar alcohols (namely, sorbitol and mannitol) differently than other sugars. These do not cause a rapid rise in blood glucose in *well-controlled* diabetes. Some physicians may therefore permit limited use of fructose by diabetic persons who are at ideal body weight and who count these calories. Because fructose has calories, overweight people should view it as little or no help in their meal plans.

The use of sugar (sucrose) in several of these recipes may seem odd. Frequently, individuals with diabetes believe they must follow a "sugar-free" diet. There is really no such diet. Milk and fruits naturally contain sugar. Breads and cereals may contain sugar as an ingredient, and breads and cereals also contain starch, a form of carbohydrate which is converted into sugar during digestion. However, use of sugar *added to food* by persons with diabetes *is usually limited,* and recipes containing sugar are used only occasionally.

Diabetic diets have traditionally been low in the amount of sucrose permitted. Use of sucrose in diabetic meal plans should be discussed with the responsible physician.

3 ☐ MEAL PLANNING AND EXCHANGES

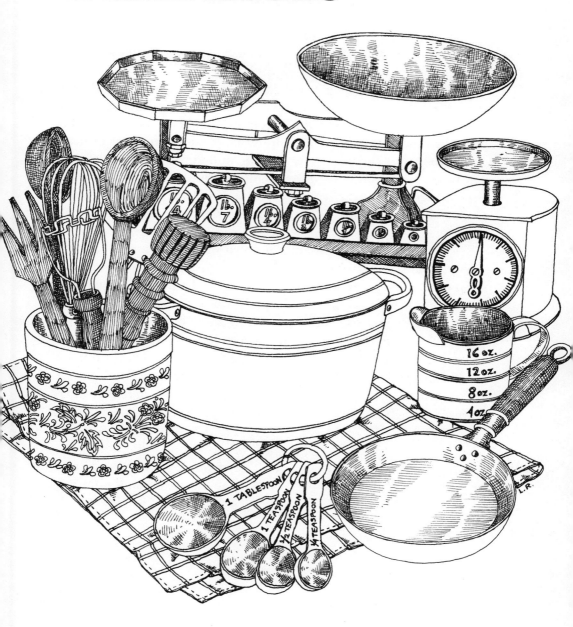

It would be an almost impossible task to calculate and balance meals that would provide all essential nutrients every day for each family member, without even considering flavor, pleasing texture, color, and economy. For these reasons, general guides have been established for various age groups, specifying the types and amounts of foods to be included in the daily diet.* Remember this rule in styling food for the family: include a wide variety of foods chosen from many different food classes.

When prescribing a diet for treatment of diabetes, a doctor considers an individual's nutritional status, weight, age, sex, daily activity, and whether or not medication is needed to help control diabetes. The diet is prescribed in terms of the number of calories and amounts of carbohydrate, protein, and fat for each day. These can be translated into a variety of meals and snacks. A daily meal plan designed by a diet counselor can be tailored to suit the individual's lifestyle, tastes, and budget. It can be altered from time to time even if the basic diet prescription remains the same.

A diet counselor is a professional with the expertise to help one plan and manage meals and food choices. A diet counselor should have special training in nutrition and dietetics and is usually a Registered Dietitian (R.D.) † Don't shortchange yourself. For competent help in an area where you need it, search out an R.D.

To obtain the help of a diet counselor ask your physician for a referral. Many communities have Registered Dietitians in private practice. Look in the yellow pages for a listing under "Dietitian" or "Nutritionist." Should you not be able to find a qualified diet counselor easily in your community, you may contact your local or

---

*The Exchange Lists and Meal Planning pattern are adapted from the *Exchange Lists for Meal Planning 1976* prepared by Committees of the American Diabetes Association, Inc., and The American Dietetic Association in cooperation with the National Institute of Arthritis, Metabolism and Digestive Diseases and the National Heart and Lung Institute, National Institutes of Health, Public Health Service, U.S. Department of Health, Education and Welfare.

† A Registered Dietitian (R.D.) has completed education and experience requirements established by The American Dietetic Association and passes an examination to demonstrate competency in dietetics, nutrition, and food service.

state American Diabetes Association Affiliate, or the district or state office of The American Dietetic Association. The Department of Dietetics of your local hospital may be able to assist you. You can also phone or write to the Director of Public Health Nutrition in the State Health or Human Resources Department in your state capital. He or she can either refer you to a Registered Dietitian near your home or provide you with some information and guidance.

A meal-planning pattern prepared by The American Diabetes and The American Dietetic Associations, and used by diet counselors, is shown in the table below. This table illustrates what a meal plan for diabetes might look like and explains how to read it. *Note : Do not use this for your meal plan.* Each person who has diabetes should have an individual plan that he or she works out with a diet counselor.

YOUR MEAL PLAN IN EXCHANGES

Must be Planned with the Assistance of Your Diet Counselor

Meal Plan for _____

Carbohydrate __250__ Protein __74__ Fat __60__ Calories 1836
        grams   grams   grams

	1 Milk	2 Veg.	3 Fruit	4 Bread	5 Meat	6 Fat
Breakfast Time 8:00 AM	1 skim	—	1½	3	—	2
Snack Time _____	—	—	—	—	—	—
Lunch or Dinner Time 12:30 PM	—	raw as desired	1	4	2 medium fat	2
Snack Time 0	—	—	—	—	—	—
Dinner or Supper Time 6:00 PM	—	1	1	3½	3 medium fat	2
Bedtime Snack Time 9:30 PM	½ skim	—	—	2	—	1

The numbers 1–6 across the top of the table refer to specific numbered Exchange Lists at the end of this chapter. Meals and snacks are identified in the left margin. The number in the box indicates how many choices to make from the specified Exchange List.

For example, follow across the middle of the chart and see what's for lunch: Raw Vegetables (list 2) and a serving of fruit or juice (list 3). The four choices from the Bread list (4) will permit two sandwiches, *each* made with two slices of whole-grain or enriched bread, 1 ounce of meat (list 5), and 1 teaspoon of mayonnaise (list 6). A noncaloric beverage of choice can be added. This is just one possible menu; your imagination is the limit.

EXCHANGES

A widely used guide for meal planning for diabetics and others who must control calories and carbohydrates is the "Exchange Lists for Meal Planning." The Exchange Lists enable people to include a wide variety of foods in what they eat each day, without having to calculate calories and balance nutrients. There are six Exchange Lists, or food classes:

1. Milk Exchanges
2. Vegetable Exchanges
3. Fruit Exchanges
4. Bread Exchanges (includes enriched or whole-grain bread, cereal, and starchy vegetables)
5. Meat Exchanges (Lean, Medium-Fat, High-Fat)
6. Fat Exchanges

Think of Exchanges as trades or options. A food within a particular Exchange List can be substituted, traded, or exchanged for another food within the *same list.* Specific size servings are indicated for each food and must be substituted in the amounts specified. Trading one food for another within one Exchange List does not significantly alter the calorie, protein, fat, and carbohydrate content of your meal plan.

The times at which meals are eaten and the intervals between them are usually determined by family members' preferences and schedules. Research has demonstrated that eating smaller amounts regularly is healthier and enables people to control their weight more easily than if they eat one or two large meals each day.

For the insulin-dependent diabetic, the number of meals and spacing are dictated by the peaking and duration of action of the insulin taken. It is crucial for the insulin-dependent diabetic to have the same number of meals and snacks each day and to eat at approximately the same times. Maintaining day-to-day consistency in amounts and distribution of carbohydrates, fats, and protein is important.

For the obese diabetic not taking insulin or oral glucose-lowering agents, regularity of meal times and consistency of meal composition are of less importance.

LIST 1 MILK EXCHANGES (Includes nonfat, low-fat, and whole milk)

One Exchange of Milk contains 12 grams of carbohydrate, 8 grams of protein, a trace of fat, and 80 calories.

Milk is a basic food for your meal plan for very good reasons. Milk is the leading source of calcium. It is a good source of phosphorus, protein, some of the B-complex vitamins, including folacin and Vitamin B_{12}, and Vitamins A and D. Magnesium is also found in milk.

Since it is a basic ingredient in many recipes, you will not find it difficult to include milk in your meal plan. Milk not only can be used to drink but can be added to cereal, coffee, tea, and other foods.

This List shows the kinds and amounts of milk or milk products to use for one Milk Exchange. Those which appear in capital letters are NONFAT. Low-fat and whole milk contain saturated fat.

NONFAT FORTIFIED MILK

SKIM OR NONFAT MILK   1 cup
POWDERED (NONFAT DRY, BEFORE ADDING LIQUID)   ⅓ cup
CANNED, EVAPORATED SKIM MILK   ½ cup
BUTTERMILK MADE FROM SKIM MILK   1 cup
YOGURT MADE FROM SKIM MILK (plain,unflavored)   1 cup

LOW-FAT FORTIFIED MILK

1% fat fortified milk (omit ½ Fat Exchange)   1 cup
2% fat fortified milk (omit 1 Fat Exchange)   1 cup
Yogurt made from 2% fortified milk (plain, unflavored) (omit 1 Fat Exchange)   1 cup

WHOLE MILK (omit 2 Fat Exchanges)

Whole milk   1 cup
Canned, evaporated whole milk   ½ cup
Buttermilk made from whole milk   1 cup
Yogurt made from whole milk (plain, unflavored)   1 cup

LIST 2 VEGETABLE EXCHANGES

One Exchange of Vegetables contains about 5 grams of carbohydrate, 2 grams of protein, and 25 calories.

The generous use of many vegetables, served either alone or in casseroles, soups, salads, or other dishes, contributes to sound health and vitality.

Dark green and deep yellow vegetables are among the leading sources of Vitamin A. Many of the vegetables in this group are also notable sources of Vitamin C: asparagus, broccoli, brussels sprouts, cabbage, cauliflower, collards, dandelion, kale, mustard and turnip greens, rutabagas, spinach, tomatoes, and turnips. A number are particularly good sources of potassium: beet greens, broccoli, brussels sprouts, chard, and tomato juice. High folacin values are found in asparagus, beets, broccoli, brussels sprouts, cauliflower, collards, kale, and lettuce. Moderate amounts of Vitamin B_6 are supplied by broccoli, brussels sprouts, cauliflower, collards, sauerkraut, spinach, tomatoes, and tomato juice. Fiber is present in all vegetables.

Whether you serve them cooked or raw, wash all vegetables even though they look clean. If fat is added in the preparation, omit the equivalent number of Fat Exchanges. The average amount of fat contained in a Vegetable Exchange that is cooked with fat meat or other fats is one Fat Exchange.

This List shows the kinds of vegetables to use for one Vegetable Exchange. One Exchange is ½ cup.

Asparagus	Greens:	Rhubarb
Bean sprouts	Beet	Rutabaga
Beets	Chards	Sauerkraut
Broccoli	Collards	String beans, green or
Brussels sprouts	Dandelion	yellow
Cabbage	Kale	Summer squash
Carrots	Mustard	Tomatoes
Cauliflower	Spinach	Tomato juice
Celery	Turnip	Turnips
Eggplant	Mushrooms	Vegetable juice
Green pepper	Okra	cocktail
	Onions	Zucchini

The following raw vegetables may be used as desired:

Chicory	Escarole	Pickles, dill
Chinese cabbage	Lettuce	Radishes
Cucumber	Parsley	Watercress
Endive		

Starchy Vegetables are found in the Bread Exchange List.

LIST 3 FRUIT EXCHANGES

One Exchange of Fruit contains 10 grams of carbohydrate and 40 calories.

Everyone likes to buy fresh fruits when they are in the height of their season. But you can also buy fresh fruits and can or freeze them for off-season use. For variety serve fruit as a salad or in combination with other foods for dessert.

Fruits are valuable for vitamins, minerals, and fiber. Vitamin C is abundant in citrus fruits and fruit juices and is found in raspberries, strawberries, mangoes, cantaloupes, honeydews, and papayas. The better sources of Vitamin A include fresh or dried apricots, mangoes, cantaloupes, nectarines, yellow peaches, and persimmons. Oranges, orange juice, and cantaloupe provide more folacin than most of the other fruits in this listing. Many fruits are a valuable source of potassium, especially apricots, bananas, several of the berries, grapefruit, grapefruit juice, mangoes, cantaloupes, honeydews, nectarines, oranges, orange juice, and peaches.

Fruit may be used fresh, dried, canned, or frozen, cooked or raw, as long as no sugar is added.

This List shows the kinds and amounts of fruits to use for one Fruit Exchange.

Apple   1 small
Apple juice   ⅓ cup
Applesauce (unsweetened)
   ½ cup
Apricots, dried   4 halves
Apricots, fresh   2 medium
Banana   ½ small
Berries
   Blackberries   ½ cup
   Blueberries   ½ cup
   Raspberries   ½ cup
   Strawberries   ¾ cup
Cherries   10 large
Cider   ⅓ cup

Dates   2
Figs, dried   1
Figs, fresh   1
Grapefruit   ½
Grapefruit juice   ½ cup
Grapes   12
Grape juice   ¼ cup
Mango   ½ small
Melon
   Cantaloupe   ¼ small
   Honeydew   ⅛ medium
   Watermelon   1 cup
Nectarine   1 small
Orange   1 small

Orange juice   ½ cup
Papaya   ¾ cup
Peach   1 medium
Pear   1 small
Persimmon, native   1 medium
Pineapple   ½ cup

Pineapple juice   ⅓ cup
Plums   2 medium
Prunes   2 medium
Prune juice   ¼ cup
Raisins   2 tablespoons
Tangerine   1 medium

Cranberries may be used as desired if no sugar is added.

LIST 4 BREAD EXCHANGES (Includes bread, cereal, and starchy vegetables)

One Exchange of Bread contains 15 grams of carbohydrate, 2 grams of protein, and 70 calories.

In this List, whole-grain and enriched breads and cereals, germ and bran products, dried beans and peas are good sources of iron and among the better sources of thiamine. The whole-grain, bran, and germ products have more fiber than products made from refined flours. Dried beans and peas are also good sources of fiber. Wheat germ, bran, dried beans, potatoes, lima beans, parsnips, pumpkin, and winter squash are particularly good sources of potassium. The better sources of folacin in this listing include whole wheat bread, wheat germ, dried beans, corn, lima beans, parsnips, green peas, pumpkin, and sweet potato.

Starchy vegetables are included in this List because they contain the same amount of carbohydrate and protein as one slice of bread.

BREAD

White (including French and
   Italian)   1 slice
Whole wheat   1 slice
Rye or pumpernickel   1 slice
Raisin   1 slice
Bagel, small   ½

English muffin, small   ½
Plain roll, bread   1
Frankfurter roll   ½
Hamburger bun   ½
Dried bread crumbs
   3 tablespoons
Tortilla, 6 inches   1

This list shows the kinds and amounts of breads, cereals, starchy vegetables, and prepared foods to use for one Bread Exchange. Those which appear in capital letters are LOW-FAT.

CEREAL

BRAN FLAKES ½ cup
OTHER READY-TO-EAT, UNSWEETENED CEREAL ¾ cup
PUFFED CEREAL (UNFROSTED) 1 cup
CEREAL (COOKED) ½ cup
GRITS (COOKED) ½ cup
RICE OR BARLEY (COOKED) ½ cup
PASTA (COOKED) ½ cup
   SPAGHETTI, NOODLES, MACARONI
POPCORN (POPPED, NO FAT ADDED, LARGE KERNEL) 3 cups
CORNMEAL (DRY) 2 tablespoons
FLOUR 2½ tablespoons
WHEAT GERM ¼ cup

CRACKERS

ARROWROOT 3
GRAHAM, 2½ inches square 2
MATZO, 4 × 6 inches ½
OYSTER 20
PRETZELS, 3⅛ inches long × ⅛ inch diameter 25
RYE WAFERS, 2 × 3½ inches 3
SALTINES 6
SODA, 2½ inch square 4

DRIED BEANS, PEAS, AND LENTILS

BEANS, PEAS, LENTILS (DRIED AND COOKED) ½ cup
BAKED BEANS, NO PORK (CANNED) ¼ cup

STARCHY VEGETABLES

CORN   ⅓ cup
CORN ON COB   1 small
LIMA BEANS   ½ cup
PARSNIPS   ⅔ cup
PEAS, GREEN (CANNED OR FROZEN)   ½ cup
POTATO, WHITE   1 small
POTATO (MASHED)   ½ cup
PUMPKIN   ¾ cup
WINTER SQUASH, ACORN OR BUTTERNUT   ½ cup
YAM OR SWEET POTATO   ¼ cup

PREPARED FOODS

Biscuit, 2 inch diameter (omit 1 Fat Exchange)   1
Corn bread, 2 × 2 × 1 inch (omit 1 Fat Exchange)   1
Corn muffin, 2 inch diameter (omit 1 Fat Exchange)   1
Crackers, round butter type (omit 1 Fat Exchange)   5
Muffin, plain small (omit 1 Fat Exchange)   1
Pancake, 5 × ½ inches (omit 1 Fat Exchange)   1
Potatoes, french fried, length 2 to 3½ inches (omit 1 Fat Exchange)   8
Potato or corn chips (omit 2 Fat Exchanges)   15
Waffle, 5 × ½ inches (omit 1 Fat Exchange)   1

LIST 5 MEAT EXCHANGES/LEAN MEAT

One Exchange of Lean Meat (1 ounce) contains 7 grams of protein, 3 grams of fat, and 55 calories.

All of the foods in the Meat Exchange Lists are good sources of protein and many are also good sources of iron, zinc, Vitamin B_{12} (present only in foods of animal origin) and other vitamins of the vitamin B-complex.

Cholesterol is of animal origin; foods of plant origin have no cholesterol.

Oysters are outstanding for their high content of zinc. Crab, liver, trimmed lean meats, the dark muscle meat of turkey, dried beans and peas, and peanut butter all have much less zinc than oysters but are still good sources.

Dried beans, peas, and peanut butter are particularly good sources of magnesium and also of potassium.

Your choice of meat groups through the week will depend on your blood lipid values. Consult with your diet counselor and your physician regarding your selection.

You may use the meat, fish, or other Meat Exchanges that are prepared for the family when no fat or flour has been added. If meat is fried, use the fat included in the meal plan. Meat juices (with the fat removed) may be used with your meat or vegetables for added flavor. Be certain to trim off all visible fat and measure meat after it has been cooked. A 3-ounce serving of cooked meat is about equal to 4 ounces of raw meat.

To plan a diet low in saturated fat and cholesterol, choose only those Exchanges in capital letters.

This List shows the kinds and amounts of lean meat and other protein-rich foods to use for one Low-Fat Meal Exchange. Trim off all visible fat.

BEEF: BABY BEEF (VERY LEAN), CHIPPED BEEF, CHUCK, FLANK STEAK, TENDERLOIN, PLATE RIBS, PLATE SKIRT STEAK, ROUND (BOTTOM, TOP), ALL CUTS RUMP, SPARE RIBS, TRIPE	1 ounce
LAMB: LEG, RIB, SIRLOIN, LOIN (ROAST AND CHOPS), SHANK, SHOULDER	1 ounce
PORK: LEG (WHOLE RUMP, CENTER SHANK), HAM, SMOKED (CENTER SLICES)	1 ounce
VEAL: LEG, LOIN, RIB, SHANK, SHOULDER, CUTLETS	1 ounce

POULTRY: CHICKEN, TURKEY, CORNISH HEN, GUINEA HEN, PHEASANT (ALL WITHOUT SKIN)	1 ounce
FISH: ANY FRESH OR FROZEN	1 ounce
CANNED SALMON, TUNA, MACKEREL, CRAB AND LOBSTER	¼ cup
CLAMS, OYSTERS, SCALLOPS, SHRIMP	5, or 1 ounce
SARDINES (DRAINED)	3
CHEESES CONTAINING LESS THAN 5% BUTTERFAT	1 ounce
COTTAGE CHEESE, DRY AND 2% BUTTERFAT	¼ cup
DRIED BEANS AND PEAS (OMIT 1 BREAD EXCHANGE)	½ cup

LIST 5 MEAT EXCHANGES/MEDIUM-FAT MEAT

One Exchange of Medium-Fat Meat (1 ounce) contains 7 grams of protein, 5 grams of fat and 75 calories.

This List shows the kinds and amounts of medium-fat meat and other protein-rich foods to use for one Medium-Fat Meat Exchange. Trim off all visible fat.

Beef: Ground (15% fat), Corned beef (canned), Rib eye, Round (ground commercial)	1 ounce
Pork: Loin (all cuts Tenderloin), Shoulder arm (picnic), Shoulder blade, Boston butt, Canadian bacon, Boiled ham	1 ounce
Liver, Heart, Kidney, and Sweetbreads (these are high in cholesterol)	1 ounce
Cottage cheese, creamed	¼ cup
Cheese: Mozzarella, Ricotta, Farmer's cheese, Neufchatel	1 ounce
Parmesan	3 tablespoons
Egg (high in cholesterol)	1
Peanut butter (omit 2 additional Fat Exchanges)	2 tablespoons

LIST 5 MEAT EXCHANGES/HIGH-FAT MEAT

One Exchange of High-Fat Meat (1 ounce) contains 7 grams of protein, 8 grams of fat and 100 calories.

This List shows the kinds and amounts of high-fat meat and other protein-rich foods to use for one High-Fat Meat Exchange. Trim off all visible fat.

Beef: Brisket, Corned beef (Brisket), Ground Beef (more than 20% fat), Hamburger (commercial), Chuck (ground commercial), Roasts (rib), Steaks (club and rib)	1 ounce
Lamb: Breast	1 ounce
Pork: Spareribs, Loin (Back ribs), Pork (ground), Country style Ham, Deviled ham	1 ounce
Veal: Breast	1 ounce
Poultry: Capon, Duck (domestic), Goose	1 ounce
Cheese: Cheddar types	1 ounce
Cold cuts	4½ × ⅛ inch slice
Frankfurter	1 small

LIST 6 FAT EXCHANGES

One Exchange of Fat contains 5 grams of fat and 45 calories.

Fats are of both animal and vegetable origin and range from liquid oils to hard fats. *Oils* are fats that remain liquid at room temperature and are usually of vegetable origin. Common fats obtained from vegetables are corn oil, olive oil, and peanut oil. Some of the common animal fats are butter and bacon fat.

Since all fats are concentrated sources of calories, foods on this List should be measured carefully to control weight. Margarine, butter, cream, and cream cheese contain Vitamin A.

This List shows the kinds and amounts of fat-containing foods to use for one Fat Exchange. To plan a diet low in saturated fats, select only those Exchanges which appear in capital letters. They are POLYUNSATURATED.

MARGARINE, SOFT, TUB OR STICK*   1 teaspoon
AVOCADO (4 inch DIAMETER)   ⅛
OIL, CORN, COTTONSEED, SAFFLOWER, SOYBEAN,
   SUNFLOWER   1 teaspoon
OIL, OLIVE †   1 teaspoon
OIL, PEANUT †   1 teaspoon
OLIVES †   5 small
ALMONDS †   10 whole
PECANS †   2 large whole
PEANUTS †
  SPANISH   20 whole
  VIRGINIA   10 whole
WALNUTS   6 small
NUTS, OTHER †   6 small

Margarine, regular stick   1 teaspoon
Butter   1 teaspoon
Bacon fat   1 teaspoon
Bacon, crisp   1 strip
Cream, light   2 tablespoons
Cream, sour   2 tablespoons
Cream, heavy   1 tablespoon
Cream cheese   1 tablespoon
French dressing ‡   1 tablespoon
Italian dressing ‡   1 tablespoon
Lard   1 teaspoon
Mayonnaise ‡   1 teaspoon
Salad dressing, mayonnaise type ‡   2 teaspoons
Salt pork   ¾-inch cube

---

*Made with corn, cottonseed, safflower, soy, or sunflower oil only.
† Fat content is primarily monounsaturated.
‡ If made with corn, cottonseed, safflower, soy, or sunflower oil, can be used in fat-modified diet.

4 □ THE OVERWEIGHT-DIABETES CONNECTION

The body needs calories to keep its inner life processes (basal metabolism) running smoothly, and for work and physical activity. Basal caloric requirements for men range from about 1600 to 1800 and for women from about 1200 to 1450 calories per day. In healthy people, the calories needed for basal metabolism are essentially the same from day to day. The number of calories required for physical activity, on the other hand, varies depending on what kind of exercise and how much is done.

With increasing age the basal metabolic rate decreases and frequently the vigor of activity does also. If the number of calories consumed is not reduced, or if physical activity is not increased, the "middle-age spread" may result.

People who are overweight stand a greater chance of developing diabetes than those who are not. About 70 percent of people with diabetes carry around too much fat.

Many overweight individuals with diabetes would have enough insulin to meet the body's needs if they returned to a normal weight. When people become too heavy, their body seems to resist insulin, so the available insulin doesn't work as well as it should.

It takes many years for obese people to develop diabetes; during this time they can make the extra insulin they need. But after some period, the insulin-producing cells (beta cells) grow tired from this extra work. They still produce insulin, but not at the same high levels. Sugar (glucose) is not removed from the blood as fast as in nondiabetic persons and accumulates, causing the symptoms of diabetes. When these people lose weight, the amount of insulin they need drops also.

Many people wonder why doctors are so concerned about weight reduction in obesity-related diabetes. The reason is that losing weight may prevent and delay complications and increase life expectancy.

WEIGHT MAINTENANCE

If the number of calories consumed is the same as the number spent, then body weight remains stable.

CALORIES IN = CALORIES OUT

A rule of thumb for estimating desirable weight for adults is as follows:

> *Women:* 100 pounds for the first 5 feet of height plus 5 pounds for each additional inch (+ 10% large frame; − 10% small frame).
>
> *Men:* 106 pounds for the first 5 feet of height plus 6 pounds for each additional inch (+ 10% large frame, − 10% small frame).

The term *obese* is often used to describe the individual who is 20 percent or more above desirable body weight.

Weight gain can result just from eating a little extra on a regular basis. A net accumulation of only 100 extra calories (either a small alcoholic drink, an ounce of meat, or a big apple) a day will result in a 10-pound weight gain in one year. A pound of fat equals about 3500 calories: when 3500 calories more than the body spends is consumed, a pound of fat is gained.

To lose a pound of fat, it is necessary to eat less than the body uses. By taking in 500 fewer calories than needed per day, a person can lose one pound in one week!

$$500 \times 7 \text{ days} = 3500$$

Obviously, since weight loss requires a calorie deficit of 3500 for each pound, reduction will be slow. But the weight wasn't gained overnight either. It is a frequent clinical observation that obese individuals eat *fewer meals* than normal-weight people. Skipping meals is not effective for long-term weight control. When meals are skipped, appetite is increased, and the tendency is to eat a bigger meal. A large amount of food overloads metabolic pathways for carbohydrate and fat, and lipogenesis is favored. Some hints for weight control are listed below:

HANDY DIET TIPS FOR CURBING CALORIES

1. Cut down on portion sizes.
2. Cut down or cut out fatty meats, fried foods, gravies, sauces, added fats, sweets, pastries, cookies, and cakes.
3. Cut down or cut out alcoholic drinks and carbonated beverages.
4. Cut down or cut out salad dressings and oils.
5. Eat more poultry and fish.
6. Drink low-fat, skim, or buttermilk.
7. Eat more fruit for dessert.
8. Eat more low-calorie vegetables.
9. Increase physical activity.

(Persons with insulin-dependent diabetes should follow their meal plan.)

25 WAYS TO THINK THIN*

1. Before you begin your diet, make a list of the reasons why you want to lose weight. While you're dieting, you can reread your reasons to help you maintain your willpower.

Diabetes Forecast, September-October 1978.

2. Keep a food diary to help you become more aware of why you overeat. Record the time and what was happening at the time. Were you watching another person eat or a TV show? Also record your feelings at the time. Were you bored, angry, or sad? See if any pattern of overeating emerges from the diary.

3. Don't weigh yourself too often. It's easy to get discouraged if you see the results on the scale every day.

4. Take a "before" picture. You'll really be able to see the difference the diet makes when you're finished losing the weight you desire. That's a great reward in itself.

5. Set reasonable goals for yourself. Weight reduction should be slow. You've had all your life to form those bad habits, so don't expect to change them all overnight. If you slip and eat something you shouldn't, don't drown yourself in disappointment by beginning a real eating binge.

6. Write out a shopping list before you go to the supermarket. Stick to the list and don't buy extra items.

7. Never go to the supermarket when you're hungry. You may be tempted to buy a lot of food you'll regret having bought when you get home.

8. Don't list too many forbidden foods for yourself. Almost all foods can be worked into a planned diet and nothing makes a food more tempting than to prohibit it altogether.

9. Don't watch TV or listen to the radio while you're eating. Without these distractions, you'll feel you're getting more out of each mouthful.

10. Chew each mouthful of food 20 times before swallowing it. It will increase your concentration on what you are eating and stretch the time you spend eating.

11. Buy yourself a present to reward yourself instead of eating. The present should have nothing to do with food, but should be clothing or some sort of entertainment.

12. Brush your teeth right after you finish eating. Once you get rid of the taste of food, you won't think about it so much.

13. Go out to a restaurant and watch other people eat. Compare how a thin person and a heavy person eat. Does the heavy person gobble down his or her food? Who looks better eating?

14. Bring a mirror to your own table and watch yourself eat.

Do you look like you're racing against time to finish your meal? Do you like the way you look as you eat?

15. Restrict your eating to one place. Don't take food into your bedroom or study. This will reduce the number of places you associate with food and eating.

16. Never skip a meal. This could be dangerous if you take insulin. Besides, most people find that if they skip one meal, they just overeat at the next.

17. Eat *before* attending a social function that features food. Then you won't be tempted to eat something you shouldn't.

18. Get more involved in family projects and community activities. Many people eat simply out of boredom and will find that other activities are much more fulfilling.

19. Take up a new hobby instead of eating. If you do sewing or woodcrafting, for instance, you'll find your hands will be busy and your mind occupied. You won't have time to think about eating.

20. Don't attach your weight loss to a specific date or event. Your goal should be long-term weight reduction and control, not losing 10 pounds to get into an Easter dress.

21. Avoid social functions that revolve around food if you feel you can't resist all the temptations.

22. Trim recipes. Make only the amount you need for one meal or place leftovers in the refrigerator before you start to eat. This cuts out the second helpings.

23. If you serve food family style (passing bowls of food around the table), serve from the kitchen range instead. Thus the food will be out of your sight and everyone else can help himself just the same.

24. Always keep food out of sight. "Out of sight, out of mind" means you may not even think about food if you're not constantly looking at it.

25. Take a walk or do some kind of exercise instead of eating. Contrary to popular belief, exercise does not increase hunger. It has the added advantage of burning calories and decreasing required insulin dosage. It also makes you feel good about yourself, something overeating never does.

5 □ EXERCISE

What is inexpensive, not fattening, fun, and good for you? Exercise! Physical activity plays an important role in health and well-being. It improves the condition of the heart, blood vessels, and lungs; improves muscle tone; helps weight loss by using energy; and lowers blood sugar.

Physical activity can be anything from a brisk walk to playing competitive handball. It can be done every day or every few days; it can be brief or sustained; it can be for work or for play. But whatever it is, it should be consistent, especially for people who take insulin. Remember that food intake, exercise, and insulin need to be balanced.

Increased exercise is an ideal way to lose a few extra pounds. It also lowers blood sugar and helps control diabetes. When diabetes is controlled by diet alone it is usually unnecessary to eat extra food before exercise. When diabetes is managed with diet and glucose-lowering pills, depending on the type and length of exercise, extra food may be required.

For people who take insulin and exercise strenuously, however, the insulin dose and the food intake must be carefully coordinated with the exercise to prevent a hypoglycemic (low blood sugar) reaction. More food, less insulin, or both may be needed. Often eating a carbohydrate-rich snack just before the exercise may be the simplest way to avoid a hypoglycemic reaction. More carbohydrate and protein snacks may be needed during and after the physical activity, depending on the kind of exercise, how long it lasts, and how intense it is. Ask your doctor and your diet counselor for more information about balancing food intake, insulin, and exercise. Here are some exercise points for anyone with diabetes:

1. Before beginning a new exercise program, talk with your doctor and have a physical checkup.
2. If you have a choice, exercise after a meal, when the blood sugar is rising, rather than before a meal.
3. If you've been living a sedentary life, start slowly.
4. Choose an exercise program or sport that you enjoy, so you will do it regularly.
5. Remember, if you use insulin, increased activity may mean you will need more food or less insulin.

Physical activity in daily living can be increased by walking to do errands; taking the stairs instead of the elevator; getting off the bus or subway a few stops early and walking; parking the car a block or two from your destination and walking. As exercise becomes more strenuous, the number of calories used increases. The number of calories used depends on body size, the kind of exercise, and the length of time and intensity of the exercise.

Being fit is now fashionable. It's also fun and healthful. Some examples of physical activity and the number of calories they burn are listed below:*

Type of Activity	Calories per Hour
Sedentary activities, such as: reading, writing; eating; watching television or movies, listening to the radio; sewing; playing cards; typing, office work, and other activities that are done while sitting and require little or no arm movement.	80 to 100
Light activities, such as: preparing and cooking food; doing dishes; dusting; handwashing small articles of clothing; ironing; walking slowly; personal care; office work and other activities that are done while standing and require some arm movement; rapid typing and other more strenuous activities done while sitting.	110 to 160

*Adapted from U.S. Department of Agriculture, Home and Garden, Bulletin No. 74. Revised 1977.

Moderate activities, such as: making beds, mopping and scrubbing; sweeping, light polishing and waxing; laundering by machine; light gardening and carpentry work; walking moderately fast; other activities that are done while standing and require moderate arm movement; activities that are done while sitting and require more vigorous arm movement.   170 to 240

Vigorous activities, such as: heavy scrubbing and waxing; handwashing large articles of clothing; hanging out clothes; stripping beds; walking fast; bowling; golfing; gardening.   250 to 350

Strenuous activities, such as: swimming; playing tennis; running; bicycling; dancing; skiing; playing football.   350 or more

6 □ RECIPES

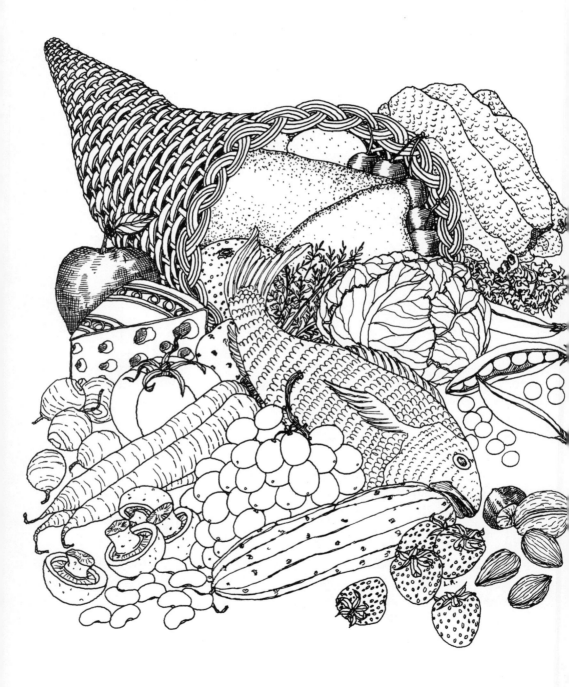

Recipes in this chapter have been kitchen-tested. However, your family's preferences, the supply of canned foods on your pantry shelf, or leftovers in your freezer may suggest many variations.

Substituting ingredients *by using foods within the same Exchange List* will not vary the recipe Exchange value for one serving, although the amounts of some nutrients, such as vitamins, may differ. Common substitutions include:

1. Turkey, tuna (water packed or well drained), or veal for chicken
2. Cauliflower or green beans for broccoli
3. Celery or green pepper for mushrooms
4. Noodles or macaroni for rice
5. Peaches for apricots

The number of variations are endless. The choice of herbs and seasonings will also vary a recipe and may increase its popularity in the family. Herbs and seasonings are "free" foods.

RECIPE SELECTION AND TESTING

To be included in the book, a recipe had to pass two tests. Each recipe was first prepared by students in the food laboratory of a college home economics department. The students and faculty formed a taste panel and judged the recipe for taste, texture, and appearance as well as the clarity of the instructions. Then each recipe was prepared in the home of a person with diabetes, who then answered questions about yield, clarity of directions, and family acceptance. The home testers represented people of all ages and included men as well as women who like to cook. Many of their thoughtful evaluations and suggestions were incorporated in the final versions of the recipes.

A WORD ABOUT THE INGREDIENTS

Milk: Skim milk is specified in the recipes. The skim milk may be fluid dairy milk, nonfat dry milk (powdered skim milk) mixed with water according to package instructions, or canned evaporated skim milk diluted with an equal measure of water.

Meats: The leanest cuts of meats and ground meat available in supermarkets were used in preparing the recipes. In addition, excess visible fat was trimmed from meats before cooking. To help keep the fat content low, the recipes indicate when fat should be drained from meats during cooking.

Broth: Recipes using beef or chicken broth may be prepared with homemade broth from which the fat has been skimmed, canned broth or bouillon, or bouillon cubes dissolved in the required amount of boiling water.

Fats: Corn, cottonseed, safflower, soybean, or sunflower oils, margarine made from these oils, and vegetable shortening are used to limit the saturated fat in the recipes. (Some vegetable fats are saturated.)

Eggs: The eggs used in all recipes are "large" eggs. We recommend that only high-quality, clean eggs with sound shells be used for recipes that call for raw or lightly cooked eggs.

Flour: Unless otherwise specified, unsifted all-purpose flour is used.

Sugar: Sugar is used in some recipes. It usually represents a small portion of the recipe's total carbohydrate content and was included when the Exchange value of the recipe was calculated. This does not mean that sugar can be sprinkled on your foods or added to beverages or used in any way except as specified in these recipes.

Ingredients, other than brown sugar and shortening, were spooned, not packed, into measuring cups and spoons.

YIELD

To help you in your meal planning, this cookbook states the anticipated yield from each recipe as clearly and accurately as possible. However, there are many reasons why the yield may vary. Differences in how finely foods are chopped, how carefully ingredients are measured, how long and at what temperature foods are simmered, the accuracy of oven thermostats, and many other factors may alter volume slightly. The total number of portions prepared from a recipe is important because *Exchange equivalents are based on single portions.*

Most of the recipes make four to six servings. A few that

serve more are particularly suitable for entertaining or for several days' use. Whenever possible, whole cans or packages of convenience foods are called for.

Recipes can be doubled for a larger group or cut down to serve one or two people. Before reducing the recipe, think about whether leftover amounts can be frozen in single-serving portions and labeled with Exchanges for use another day.

When deciding to prepare a recipe, note the size of the serving. A yield of six half-cup servings may feed only four people if one of the people is a hungry teenager.

Remember, this book is not a basic how-to-cook cookbook. It does not tell you how to broil a steak, roast a turkey, or boil vegetables. Rather, it offers recipes you may have avoided because you did not know the Exchange values.

"EXCHANGES" AND "ESTIMATED NUTRIENTS" PER SERVING

For each recipe, the Exchanges and the estimated value for energy (calories) grams of carbohydrate, protein, fat, and milligrams of sodium and potassium are listed for one serving. The nutrients per serving are expressed in abbreviations and symbols as follows:

Calories   CAL
Carbohydrates   CHO
Protein   PRO
Fat   FAT
Sodium   Na
Potassium   K
Not available   NA

To guarantee the exact energy and nutrient values of foods eaten would require a laboratory installed in each home. The nutrient composition of foods is influenced by the location from which the food comes, the season, degree of ripeness, preparation for market, home storage, and preparation for the table. Therefore, the nutritional information is approximate.

The Exchanges and nutrients per serving were derived from the Exchange Lists, food tables, computer data, and product information. Note that sodium and potassium estimates are not included for recipe ingredients listed "as desired," "dash," or "to taste."

Appetizers

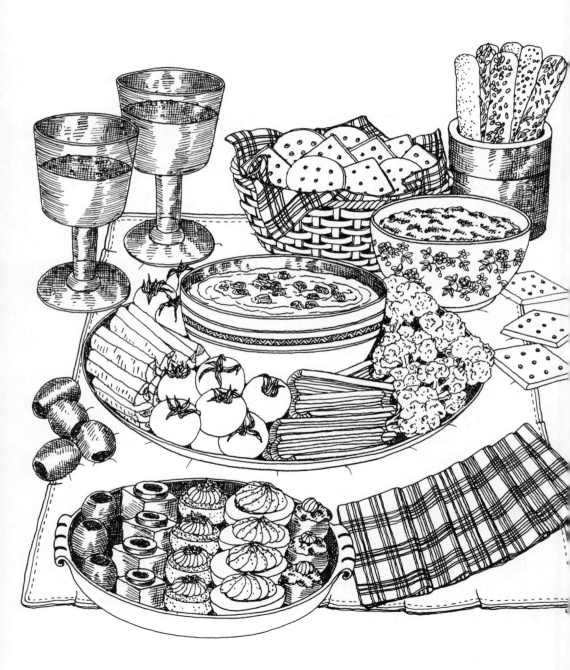

Appetizers, dips, and such are usually served when company comes. They keep the guests busily occupied while the hostess completes meal preparations.

The appetizer board may be very simple, with two or three crisp vegetables to nibble, a bowl of dip, and perhaps some crisp wafers, pretzels, or cheese sticks. A tomato juice cocktail or cup of bouillon could be served as beverage.

Vegetables for dips may include cucumber fingers, either peeled or with skin on, carrot sticks, celery, radishes, scallions, cauliflower buds, green pepper slices or rings, all chilled and crisp. The list is endless.

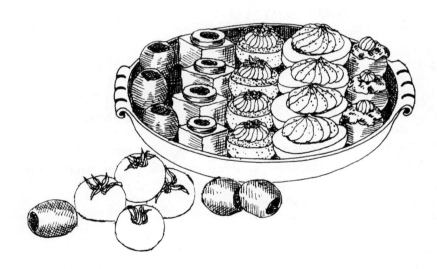

Cocktail Ham Balls

Yield: 48 balls (12 servings)
Exchanges per 4 balls serving:
   1 High-Fat Meat
   ½ Vegetable
   1 Fat

Estimated nutrients per serving:

CAL	157	FAT	13
CHO	2	Na	190
PRO	8	K	111

Ingredients

  ½ POUND BULK PORK SAUSAGE
  2 CUPS COOKED HAM, GROUND (ABOUT ½ POUND)
  ¼ CUP CHOPPED GREEN ONIONS WITH TOPS
  1 5-OUNCE CAN WATER CHESTNUTS, DRAINED AND FINELY CHOPPED
  1 EGG
  1 TABLESPOON SKIM MILK
  1 GARLIC CLOVE, CRUSHED

Method

1. Brown sausage. Drain all excess fat.
2. Mix all ingredients. Form into 4 dozen balls, using 2 teaspoons meat per ball.
3. Brown slowly in pan coated with vegetable pan spray.
4. Lower heat; continue cooking 10 minutes or until meat is entirely cooked.
5. Serve hot with toothpicks.

Marinated Mushrooms

Yield: 2 cups (4 servings)
Exchanges per ½-cup serving
   ½ Vegetable
   2 Fat

Estimated nutrients per serving:
CAL	97	FAT	9
CHO	3	Na	272
PRO	1	K	21

Ingredients

    1 CUP WATER
    ⅓ CUP VEGETABLE OIL
    ⅓ CUP LEMON JUICE
    1 GARLIC CLOVE, PEELED AND CRUSHED
    ½ TEASPOON THYME
    ½ TEASPOON TARRAGON
    1 TEASPOON SALT
    ½ TEASPOON PEPPERCORNS
    2 6-OUNCE CANS MUSHROOM CROWNS, DRAINED

Method

1. Combine all ingredients except mushrooms in saucepan. Simmer uncovered 5 minutes.
2. Add mushrooms; simmer 1 minute.
3. Cover; refrigerate, stirring several times.
4. Serve drained, with toothpicks.

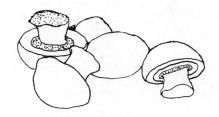

Blue Cheese Dip

Yield: 2 cups (16 servings)

Exchanges per 2-tablespoon serving:

    ½ Medium-Fat Meat

Estimated nutrients per serving:

CAL	42	FAT	3
CHO	1	Na	160*
PRO	3	K	43

Ingredients

  1 CUP LOW-FAT COTTAGE CHEESE
  ½ CUP PLAIN, LOW-FAT YOGURT
  4 OUNCES BLUE CHEESE, CRUMBLED
    DASH ONION SALT*
    DASH WORCESTERSHIRE SAUCE
    DASH TABASCO SAUCE

Method

1. Puree cottage cheese with yogurt in blender if smooth dip is desired.
2. Combine with remaining ingredients. Refrigerate.
3. Serve with raw vegetables or crisp crackers.

*Na content of onion salt not included in estimate.

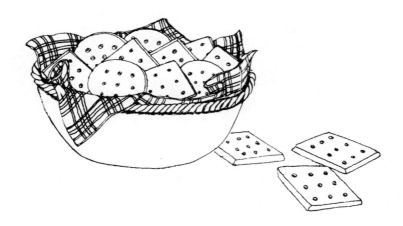

Creamy Onion Dip

Yield: 1 cup (8 servings)
Exchanges per 2-tablespoon
serving:

    ½ Vegetable
    1 Fat

Estimated nutrients per serving:

CAL	66	FAT	6
CHO	2	Na	102
PRO	1	K	44

Ingredients

    2 TABLESPOONS DRY ONION SOUP MIX
    1 CUP DAIRY SOUR CREAM

Method

1. Stir onion soup mix into sour cream.
2. Chill. Serve with vegetable relish tray.

Cheddar Cheese Dip

Yield: 1 cup (16 servings)
Exchanges per 1-tablespoon
serving:

    ½ Fat

Estimated nutrients per serving:

CAL	24	FAT	2
CHO	1	Na	97
PRO	1	K	29

Ingredients

    ½ CUP GRATED CHEDDAR CHEESE (ABOUT 2 OUNCES)
    1 6-OUNCE CARTON PLAIN, LOW-FAT YOGURT
    ½ TEASPOON SALT
    2 TABLESPOONS MINCED FRESH PARSLEY

Method

1. Combine all ingredients. Blend well.
2. Chill 6 to 8 hours.
3. Serve with cauliflower, celery, or other crisp raw vegetables.

Spicy Vegetable Dip

Yield: 1⅓ cups (12 servings)
Exchanges per 2-tablespoon
serving:
    Free

Estimated nutrients per serving:

CAL	20	FAT	1
CHO	3	Na	315
PRO	1	K	74

Ingredients

  1 8-OUNCE CARTON PLAIN, LOW-FAT YOGURT
¼ CUP CHILI SAUCE
  1 TABLESPOON PREPARED HORSERADISH
  1 TEASPOON GRATED LEMON RIND
  1 TEASPOON SALT
  2 TABLESPOONS MINCED CELERY
  1 TABLESPOON MINCED GREEN PEPPER
  1 TABLESPOON MINCED GREEN ONION

Method

1. Combine all ingredients. Mix well.
2. Chill thoroughly.
3. Serve as a dip for celery sticks, green onions, green pepper, cauliflower, and other crisp raw vegetables.

Onion Sticks

Yield: 96 sticks (16 servings)
Exchanges per 6-stick serving:
    1 Bread
    1½ Fat

Estimated nutrients per serving:

CAL	135	FAT	7
CHO	16	Na	383
PRO	2	K	50

Ingredients

  1 1½-OUNCE ENVELOPE DRY ONION SOUP MIX
¼ POUND (½ CUP) MARGARINE, SOFTENED
16 SLICES SANDWICH BREAD

Method

1. Preheat oven to 375° F.
2. Combine soup mix with margarine. Mix with fork.
3. Spread mixture on bread, using about 1½ teaspoons per slice.
4. Cut each slice into 6 sticks. Place in single layer on large baking sheet.
5. Bake for 8 to 10 minutes until brown and crisp.

Hints: Fresh bread is easier to spread and slice if partially frozen. Leftover sticks may be stored in tightly closed container.

Cheese Sticks

Yield: 96 sticks (16 servings)
Exchanges per 6-stick serving
    1 Bread
    1½ Fat

Estimated nutrients per serving:

CAL	135	FAT	7
CHO	15	Na	243
PRO	3	K	31

Ingredients

½ CUP GRATED PARMESAN CHEESE
¼ POUND (½ CUP) MARGARINE, SOFTENED
16 SLICES SANDWICH BREAD
    PAPRIKA AS DESIRED (OPTIONAL)

Method

1. Preheat oven to 375° F.
2. With fork, combine cheese with margarine.
3. Spread mixture on bread, using about 1½ teaspoons per slice.
4. Sprinkle with paprika, if desired.
5. Cut each slice into 6 sticks. Place in single layer on large baking sheet.
6. Bake for 8 to 10 minutes until brown and crisp.

Sesame-Cheese Wafers

Yield: 24 wafers (6 servings)
Exchanges per 4-wafer serving:
    1 Bread
    1 High-Fat Meat

Estimated nutrients per serving:

CAL	157	FAT	9
CHO	13	Na	351
PRO	6	K	85

Ingredients

- 2 TABLESPOONS SESAME SEEDS
- 1 5-OUNCE JAR PROCESSED SHARP CHEESE SPREAD
- 4 TEASPOONS MARGARINE
- ¾ CUP SIFTED FLOUR
- ¼ TEASPOON PAPRIKA

Method

1. Preheat oven to 350° F.
2. Toast sesame seeds in pie pan in oven for 5 to 10 minutes, stirring once to brown evenly.
3. In small bowl cream together cheese spread and margarine.
4. Add flour, paprika, and sesame seeds. Mix thoroughly.
5. Form into a 6-inch-long roll. Wrap in foil. Refrigerate. (Dough may be refrigerated for up to 1 week.)
6. When ready to bake, preheat oven to 400° F. Slice roll into ¼-inch wafers.
7. Bake on ungreased baking sheet 8 to 10 minutes or until edges are lightly browned. Remove from baking sheet. Cool.

Cereal Party Mix

Yield: 4 cups (8 servings)
Exchanges per ½-cup serving:

    1 Bread

    1 Fat

Estimated nutrients per serving:

CAL	92	FAT	4
CHO	13	Na	203
PRO	1	K	17

Ingredients

   2 TABLESPOONS MARGARINE
  ½ TEASPOON SEASONED SALT
   2 TEASPOONS WORCESTERSHIRE SAUCE
   1 CUP RICE CHEX
1½ CUPS WHEAT CHEX
   1 CUP THIN PRETZEL STICKS (1 OUNCE, OR ABOUT 90 STICKS)
  ½ CUP CHEESE TIDBITS (1 OUNCE, OR ABOUT 32 CRACKERS)

Method

1. Preheat oven to 250° F.
2. Melt margarine in shallow baking pan. Stir in salt and Worcestershire sauce.
3. Add remaining ingredients. Stir to coat pieces with margarine.
4. Heat 45 minutes, stirring every 15 minutes.
5. Spread on paper toweling to cool. Store in tight container.

Suggestion: Measure ½-cup portions into paper cups for a party appetizer or snack.

Soups

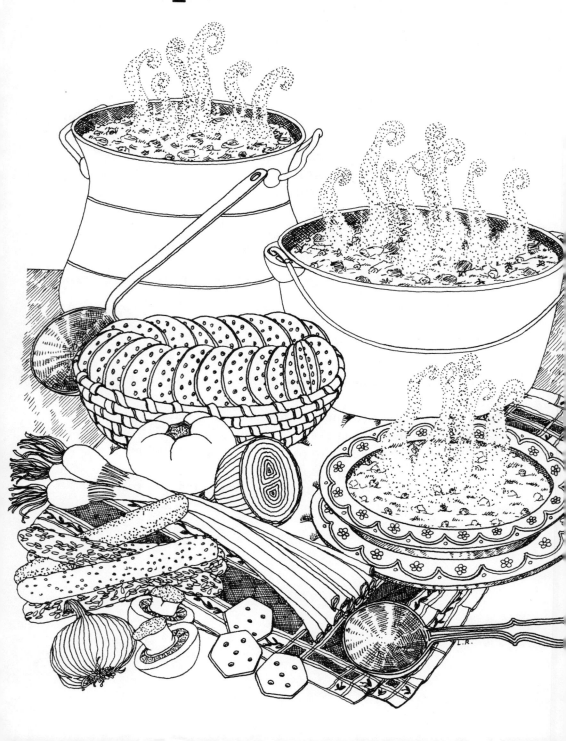

Soups are versatile. A hearty soup, such as one of the chowders, can be almost a meal in itself. Other soups may serve as first course at dinner or part of a soup-sandwich-fruit lunch. They can cool you on a warm day (gazpacho, for example) or warm you on a chilly day. Some of these soups may provide a way to introduce new vegetables to your family.

Garnishes for soups may include a few croutons; a floating teaspoonful of sour cream, chopped chives, or parsley; or mushroom slices. Crackers, bread sticks, or crusty rolls go well with soup. See the Appetizer and Bread chapters for additional suggestions.

Spicy Tomato Bouillon

Yield: 3 cups (3 servings)
Exchanges per 1-cup serving:
   2 Vegetable

Estimated nutrients per serving:

CAL	52	FAT	—
CHO	8	Na	972
PRO	5	K	442

Ingredients

1¾ CUPS TOMATO JUICE
  1 10½-OUNCE CAN CONDENSED BEEF BROTH
  1 TEASPOON LEMON JUICE
¼ TEASPOON WORCESTERSHIRE SAUCE
¼ TEASPOON HORSERADISH

Method

1. Combine all ingredients in medium saucepan.
2. Simmer for approximately 10 minutes.
3. Serve hot.

Tomato Rice Broth

Yield: 2⅔ cups (2 servings)
Exchanges per 1⅓-cup serving:
2 Bread

Estimated nutrients per serving:

CAL	136	FAT	—
CHO	28	Na	1732
PRO	6	K	281

Ingredients

½ CUP TOMATO JUICE
1¾ CUPS CLEAR BEEF OR CHICKEN BROTH
1 CUP COOKED RICE
½ TEASPOON SALT
PEPPER TO TASTE

Method

1. Combine all ingredients in saucepan.
2. Bring to boil. Serve.

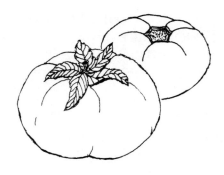

French Onion Soup

Yield: 6 cups (6 servings)
Exchanges per 1-cup serving:
    1 Vegetable
    ½ Bread
    1 Fat

Estimated nutrients per serving:

CAL	113	FAT	5
CHO	12	Na	892
PRO	5	K	252

Ingredients

   4 LARGE ONIONS, THINLY SLICED
   2 TABLESPOONS MARGARINE
4½ CUPS BEEF BROTH
   1 TEASPOON WORCESTERSHIRE SAUCE
  ½ TEASPOON SALT
  ⅛ TEASPOON PEPPER
   2 SLICES FRENCH BREAD, TOASTED
   2 TABLESPOONS GRATED PARMESAN CHEESE

Method

1. Saute onions in margarine until lightly browned.
2. Add broth, Worcestershire sauce, salt, and pepper.
3. Simmer 20 minutes.
4. Sprinkle toast with Parmesan cheese; place under broiler a few seconds until cheese is browned. Cut each slice into 3 pieces.
5. Pour soup in bowls and float toast slices on top.

French Vegetable Soup

Yield: 6 cups (6 servings)
Exchanges per 1-cup serving:
    1 Vegetable
    1 Bread
    1 Fat

Estimated nutrients per serving:

CAL	145	FAT	5
CHO	19	Na	743*
PRO	6	K	577

Ingredients

  10 GREEN ONIONS, SLICED
1½ CUPS CHOPPED CELERY
  1 TABLESPOON MARGARINE
1½ CUPS CHOPPED CARROT
1½ CUPS CUBED TURNIP
4½ CUPS CHICKEN STOCK
  ¼ TEASPOON THYME
     SALT* AND PEPPER AS DESIRED
1½ CUPS COOKED GREAT NORTHERN BEANS
  6 TABLESPOONS DAIRY SOUR CREAM

Method

1. Saute onion and celery in margarine until tender.
2. Add remaining ingredients except beans and sour cream. Simmer until vegetables are tender.
3. Add beans. (Beans may be pureed in blender if desired.)
4. Heat through. Garnish each serving with 1 tablespoon sour cream.

*Na content of salt not included in estimate.

Oyster Stew

Yield: 2 cups (2 servings)
Exchanges per 1-cup serving:

    2 Lean Meat
    1 Bread
    ½ Fat

Estimated nutrients per serving:

CAL	201	FAT	9
CHO	15	Na	690
PRO	15	K	330

Ingredients

  1 TABLESPOON MARGARINE
  1 TABLESPOON FLOUR
  1 CUP SKIM MILK
  ½ TEASPOON SALT
  ½ TEASPOON WORCESTERSHIRE SAUCE
    DASH OF HOT PEPPER SAUCE
  1 CUP OYSTERS, SHUCKED, UNDRAINED (ABOUT ½ PINT)
  2 TABLESPOONS MINCED FRESH PARSLEY

Method

1. Melt margarine. Remove from heat.
2. Using a French whip, gradually add flour, mixing until smooth. Add milk, stirring.
3. Heat slowly; continue mixing until thickened.
4. Add salt, Worcestershire sauce, and hot pepper sauce.
5. In a separate pot, simmer oysters in their own juice just until edges curl.
6. Add oysters and juice to white sauce. Heat through.
7. Garnish with parsley.

Cream of Mushroom Soup

Yield: 4 cups (4 servings)

Exchanges per 1-cup serving:
    ½ Milk
    ½ Vegetable

Estimated nutrients per serving:

CAL	61	FAT	1
CHO	9	Na	565
PRO	5	K	159

Ingredients

  2 8-OUNCE CANS MUSHROOMS, DRAINED AND MINCED
1½ CUPS CHICKEN BROTH (OR 1 13-OUNCE CAN READY-
    TO-SERVE)
1½ CUPS SKIM MILK
  ½ TEASPOON SALT
    PEPPER TO TASTE
  ½ TEASPOON WORCESTERSHIRE SAUCE

Method

1. Simmer mushrooms in broth 15 minutes.
2. Add remaining ingredients and simmer 15 minutes.

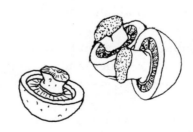

Potato Soup

Yield: 5 cups (4 servings)
Exchanges per 1¼-cup serving:
  ½ Milk
  1 Bread

Estimated nutrients per serving:

CAL	105	FAT	1
CHO	20	Na	1176
PRO	6	K	464

Ingredients

  2 CUPS PEELED, DICED POTATOES
  ½ CUP MINCED ONION
  1 13¾-OUNCE CAN CHICKEN BROTH
  1 TEASPOON SALT
  ½ TEASPOON CELERY SALT
  ⅛ TEASPOON PEPPER
  2 CUPS SKIM MILK
  1 TABLESPOON MINCED CHIVES

Method

1. Put all ingredients except milk and chives in saucepan and simmer, covered, until potatoes are tender, about 15 minutes.
2. Add milk. Simmer uncovered 5 minutes.
3. Garnish with chives.

Cream of Cauliflower Soup

Yield: 6 cups (6 servings)

Exchanges per 1-cup serving:
   ½ Milk
   1 Medium-Fat Meat
   2 Vegetable
   1 Fat

Estimated nutrients per serving:

CAL	210	FAT	10
CHO	15	Na	596
PRO	15	K	527

Ingredients

  1 10-OUNCE PACKAGE FROZEN CAULIFLOWER
  1 10¾-OUNCE CAN CONDENSED CHICKEN BROTH, DIVIDED
  ½ TEASPOON MACE
  1 10-OUNCE PACKAGE FROZEN CHOPPED BROCCOLI
  ½ TEASPOON MUSTARD SEED
  ½ TEASPOON DILL WEED
  ⅓ CUP CHOPPED ONION
  2 TABLESPOONS MARGARINE
  2 TABLESPOONS FLOUR
  ½ TEASPOON SALT
    DASH OF PEPPER
3¾ CUPS SKIM MILK
  1 CUP SHREDDED SWISS CHEESE (ABOUT 4 OUNCES)

Method

1. Cook cauliflower, covered, in ½ cup broth for 5 to 8 minutes or until tender. Do not drain. Process in blender with mace until smooth.
2. Cook broccoli, covered, in remaining broth with mustard seed and dill weed for 5 to 8 minutes or until tender.

3. Saute onion in margarine until tender. Add flour, salt, and pepper. Add milk. Cook, stirring, until thickened.
4. Add cauliflower and broccoli mixtures and cheese to sauce. Cook and stir until just heated through and cheese is melted.

Variation: Substitute different vegetables for cauliflower and broccoli. For example, try pureed spinach and chopped carrots or turnips for contrast.

Fish Chowder

Yield: 4½ cups (6 servings)
Exchanges per ¾-cup serving:
    ½ Milk
    1 Lean Meat
    ½ Vegetable
    ½ Fat

Estimated nutrients per serving:

CAL	134	FAT	6
CHO	10	Na	282
PRO	10	K	418

Ingredients

  2 SLICES BACON, CHOPPED
½ CUP CHOPPED ONION
½ CUP WATER
  1 CUP DICED POTATOES
  1 POUND WHITEFISH FILLETS, DICED
  2 CUPS SKIM MILK
½ TEASPOON SALT
   PEPPER TO TASTE
  1 TABLESPOON CHOPPED FRESH PARSLEY

Method

1. Cook bacon until crisp. Add onion and brown slightly. Drain fat.
2. Add water and potato. Cook about 10 minutes until potatoes are partially tender.
3. Add fish. Continue cooking until fish can be flaked with a fork.
4. Add milk, salt, and pepper, and heat.
5. Serve in bowls; sprinkle with parsley.

Frank and Corn Chowder

Yield: 4 cups (4 servings)
Exchanges per 1-cup serving:

   2 High-Fat Meat
   2 Bread
   2 Fat

Estimated nutrients per serving:

CAL	421	FAT	25
CHO	30	Na	1110
PRO	19	K	422

Ingredients

  ½ POUND FRANKFURTERS, HALVED LENGTHWISE AND SLICED
  ½ CUP CHOPPED GREEN PEPPER
  ½ CUP CHOPPED ONION
  1 17-OUNCE CAN CREAM-STYLE CORN
  ¾ CUP SKIM MILK
  1 CUP CUBED CHEDDAR CHEESE (ABOUT 4 OUNCES)

Method

1. Saute franks, green pepper, and onion in saucepan sprayed with vegetable pan spray.
2. Add remaining ingredients; stir until cheese melts.
3. Serve hot.

Greek Lentil Soup

Yield: 8 cups (8 servings)
Exchanges per 1-cup serving:
    1 Lean Meat
    1½ Bread

Estimated nutrients per serving:

CAL	156	FAT	4
CHO	22	Na	424
PRO	8	K	401

Ingredients

1¼ CUPS LENTILS (ABOUT ½ POUND)
  1 QUART COLD WATER
  1 CUP CHOPPED ONION
  1 GARLIC CLOVE, CRUSHED
1¼ TEASPOONS SALT
 ¼ TEASPOON PEPPER
  2 TABLESPOONS VEGETABLE OIL
  1 16-OUNCE CAN TOMATOES
  1 BAY LEAF

Method

1. Wash lentils; drain well.
2. Combine lentils with water, onion, garlic, salt, pepper, and oil in large saucepan. Bring to boil. Add tomatoes and bay leaf.
3. Lower heat; cover and simmer 45 minutes or until lentils are tender.
4. Serve with lemon juice or wine vinegar if desired.

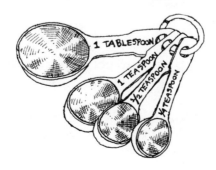

Hearty Split Pea Soup

Yield: 8 cups (8 servings)
Exchanges per 1-cup serving:

    1 Lean Meat
    1 Vegetable
    2 Bread

Estimated nutrients per serving:

CAL	206	FAT	2
CHO	35	Na	597
PRO	12	K	522

Ingredients

    2 CUPS SPLIT PEAS
    1 HAM BONE
    6 CUPS WATER
    1 CUP CHOPPED CARROT
    ½ CUP CHOPPED ONION
    ½ CUP CHOPPED CELERY
    1 TABLESPOON MARGARINE
    ¼ CUP CHOPPED CELERY LEAVES
    2 TABLESPOONS CHOPPED FRESH PARSLEY (OR
      1 TABLESPOON PARSLEY FLAKES)
    2 TEASPOONS SALT
    1 TEASPOON BASIL
    ¼ TEASPOON ALLSPICE
    ¼ TEASPOON THYME
    1 BAY LEAF
    2 CUPS CHOPPED RAW SPINACH
    1 CUP FROZEN GREEN PEAS

Method

1. Place split peas in large soup pot with ham bone. Add water.
2. Saute carrots, onion, and celery in margarine until tender. Add to peas.
3. Add remaining ingredients except spinach and green peas. Bring to boil; cover and simmer 30 minutes.

4. Add spinach and green peas. Simmer 30 more minutes.
5. Remove ham bone and bay leaf.

Variation: After cooking, soup may be pureed in blender if smooth consistency is preferred.

Gazpacho

Yield: 4 cups (4 servings)
Exchanges per 1-cup serving:
    1 Vegetable
   1½ Fat

Estimated nutrients per serving:

CAL	103	FAT	7
CHO	8	Na	588
PRO	2	K	514

Ingredients

4 MEDIUM TOMATOES, QUARTERED
1 SMALL CUCUMBER, PEELED AND SLICED
¼ CUP SLICED ONION
2 STALKS CELERY, QUARTERED
½ GREEN PEPPER, SLICED
1 CLOVE GARLIC, MINCED
1 TEASPOON SALT
¼ TEASPOON PEPPER
2 TABLESPOONS SALAD OIL
3 TABLESPOONS WINE VINEGAR
½ CUP ICE WATER

Method

1. Core and remove seeds from 1 tomato. Chop finely. Set aside.
2. Combine all other ingredients in blender container. Blend only a few *seconds*. Mixture should *not* be smooth.
3. Add chopped tomato. Chill.
4. Serve in chilled bowls with an ice cube in each serving.

Cucumber Soup

Yield: 3 cups (4 servings)
Exchanges per ¾-cup serving:
   ½ Milk
    1 Vegetable
    1 Fat

Estimated nutrients per serving:

CAL	122	FAT	6
CHO	12	Na	387
PRO	5	K	300

Ingredients

- 2 TABLESPOONS MARGARINE
- 2 TABLESPOONS FLOUR
- 1 CUP CHICKEN BROTH
- 1 CUP EVAPORATED SKIM MILK
- 2 TABLESPOONS CHOPPED FRESH CHIVES
- 2 TABLESPOONS CHOPPED CELERY LEAVES
- 2 TABLESPOONS CHOPPED FRESH PARSLEY
- 1 LARGE CUCUMBER, PEELED
- 2 TABLESPOONS WATER

Method

1. Melt margarine in saucepan over low heat. Blend in flour.
2. Slowly add broth and milk, stirring constantly. Cook, stirring, until smooth and thickened.
3. Stir in chives, celery, and parsley. Remove from heat.
4. Puree cucumber in blender with 2 tablespoons water. Slowly stir into sauce.
5. Heat until just warm or serve chilled. Excessive heat may cause soup to curdle.

Chicken Egg Drop Soup

Yield: 4 cups (4 servings)
Exchanges per 1-cup serving:
½ Medium-Fat Meat

Estimated nutrients per serving:

CAL	34	FAT	2
CHO	1	Na	996
PRO	3	K	77

Ingredients

- 1 TABLESPOON DICED ONION
- ½ CUP CHOPPED CELERY
- 4 CUPS CHICKEN BROTH
- 1 EGG, SLIGHTLY BEATEN

Method

1. Cook onion and celery in broth until tender.
2. Slowly pour beaten egg into boiling broth, stirring so egg separates into shreds.

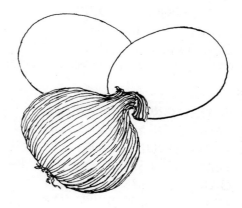

Vegetable and Meatball Soup

Yield: 5 cups (4 servings)
Exchanges per 1¼-cup,
2 meatball serving:

    3 Lean Meat
    1 Bread
    1 Fat

Estimated nutrients per serving:

CAL	269	FAT	13
CHO	17	Na	NA
PRO	21	K	NA

Ingredients

  ½ MEDIUM ONION, CHOPPED
  1 MEDIUM CARROT, CHOPPED
  ½ CUP CHOPPED CELERY
  1 TABLESPOON VEGETABLE OIL
  1 MEDIUM TOMATO, PEELED AND CHOPPED
  ¼ TEASPOON GROUND GINGER
  ¼ TEASPOON CUMIN
  ¼ TEASPOON PAPRIKA
  1 TABLESPOON CHOPPED FRESH PARSLEY
  1 QUART BEEF BROTH
  ¼ CUP TOMATO SAUCE
  ¼ CUP DRY LENTILS (UNCOOKED)

Meatballs
  ½ POUND GROUND LAMB
  3 TABLESPOONS BEEF STOCK
  1 TABLESPOON FLOUR
  ½ TEASPOON SALT
  1 GARLIC CLOVE, CRUSHED
  1 TEASPOON CHOPPED PARSLEY

Method

1. Saute onion, carrot, and celery in oil until tender.
2. Add remaining ingredients except meatballs. Simmer 30 minutes.
3. Make 8 meatballs with remaining ingredients. Add to soup. Simmer 15 minutes or until meat is done.

Pinto Bean Soup

Yield: 6 cups (6 servings)
Exchanges per 1-cup serving:
    2 Medium-Fat Meat
    1 Bread
    ½ Fat

Estimated nutrients per serving:

CAL	250	FAT	14
CHO	15	Na	NA
PRO	16	K	NA

Ingredients

⅝ CUP (4 OUNCES) PINTO BEANS
3 CUPS WATER
1 POUND BEEF SHANKS
½ MEDIUM ONION, SLICED
½ TEASPOON SALT
⅛ TEASPOON THYME
1 BAY LEAF
1 MEDIUM CARROT, DICED

Method

1. Place beans in large soup pot with water. Boil 2 minutes; cover; remove from heat; let stand 1 hour.
2. Cut meat into small cubes. Brown slowly in skillet with onion.
3. Add shank bones and remaining ingredients, except carrots, to beans. Simmer 1 hour or until beans are tender. Remove bones and bay leaf.
4. Add carrot. Simmer 30 minutes or until tender.

Main Dishes:
Meats

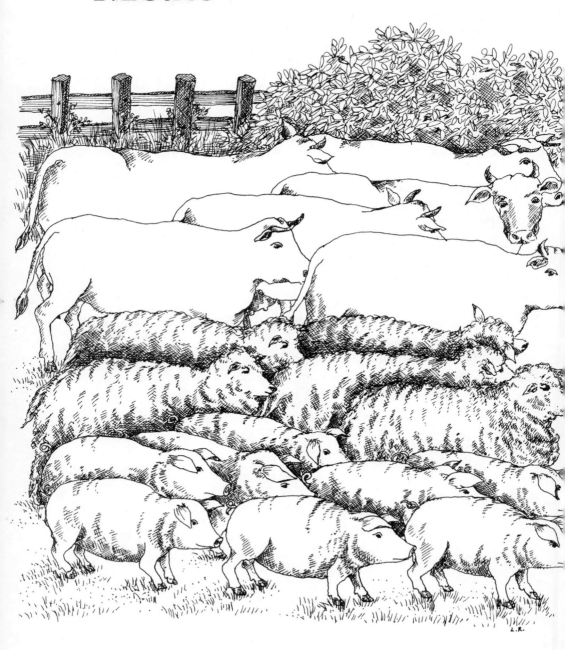

This section includes beef, veal, lamb, and pork dishes. Many of the recipes use ground beef or leftover cooked meats. To keep fat exchanges to a minimum, select the leaner cuts or packages of meats when shopping. Trim off visible fat, and always drain excess fat when browning ground meat.

The one-dish meals in this section are easy to prepare and can go to the table in the baking dish. The basic ingredients should be measured accurately. You may vary seasonings to suit your family's taste. Ingredients such as onion, green pepper, mushrooms, and celery may be increased, decreased, or interchanged with only a small variation in the recipe's yield or exchanges.

If you're in the mood, try preparing tacos, sloppy joes, or individual pizzas for the family.

Swiss Steak

Yield: 6 servings
Exchanges per 1/6 recipe serving:

2 Lean Meat
1 Vegetable
½ Bread

Estimated nutrients per serving:

CAL	161	FAT	5
CHO	13	Na	649
PRO	16	K	518

Ingredients

- ¼ CUP FLOUR
- 1 TEASPOON SALT
- ¼ TEASPOON PEPPER
- 1 POUND BEEF ROUND STEAK, ABOUT ¾ INCH THICK
- 1 TABLESPOON VEGETABLE OIL
- 1 LARGE ONION, SLICED
- 1 16-OUNCE CAN TOMATOES
- ½ CUP BEEF BROTH
- 2 CUPS PEELED, SLICED CARROT

Method

1. Combine flour, salt, and pepper. Coat steak with seasoned flour.
2. With wooden mallet pound meat between wax paper until it's ½ inch thick. Cut into 6 serving pieces.
3. Heat oil in large skillet.
4. Brown steak well on both sides. Move to one side of skillet to saute onion until tender.
5. Add tomatoes and broth.
6. Cover and simmer 1½ hours.
7. Add carrots, cover, simmer ½ hour, or until meat and carrots are tender.

Beef Burgundy

Yield: 4 cups (8 servings)
Exchanges per ½-cup serving:
    2½ Lean Meat
      1 Vegetable

Estimated nutrients per serving:

CAL	153	FAT	5
CHO	5	Na	440
PRO	22	K	407

Ingredients

    2 POUNDS TOP ROUND STEAK
    1 3-OUNCE CAN MUSHROOMS, SLICED
    1 TABLESPOON FLOUR
    1 ENVELOPE DRY ONION SOUP MIX
1¾ CUPS WATER
 ½ CUP DRY RED WINE

Method

1. Preheat oven to 350° F.
2. Cut steak into 1-inch cubes.
3. Brown meat slowly in skillet sprayed with vegetable pan spray. Transfer to 1½-quart casserole which has tight-fitting cover.
4. Add remaining ingredients. Stir well.
5. Cover and bake for 1½ hours.
6. Remove cover and bake 15 minutes longer or until tender.

Serving suggestion: Serve on toast, rice, or noodles. Remember to add the Bread Exchanges.

Oven Meatballs

Yield: 48 meatballs (8 servings)
Exchanges per 6-meatball
serving:

  2 Medium-Fat Meat
  ½ Bread
  ½ Fat

Estimated nutrients per serving:

CAL	222	FAT	14
CHO	6	Na	379
PRO	18	K	345

Ingredients

  ½ CUP SKIM MILK
  ¼ CUP FINELY CHOPPED ONION
  2 EGGS
  1 TEASPOON SALT
  3 SLICES BREAD, CRUMBLED
  1½ POUNDS GROUND BEEF

Method

1. Preheat oven to 375° F.
2. Combine milk, onion, eggs, and salt. Add bread crumbs; let stand for 5 minutes.
3. Add meat and mix thoroughly.
4. Shape into 4 dozen small balls 1 to 1½ inches in diameter.
5. Place on baking pan and bake for 20 to 30 minutes.

Serving suggestion: May be used with Spaghetti Sauce or Stroganoff Sauce (see next two recipes).
Meatballs may be frozen in serving sizes in plastic bags for future use.

Oven Meatballs in Stroganoff Sauce

Yield: 2 cups sauce (4 servings)
Exchanges per ½-cup sauce and
6-meatball serving:

    2 Medium-Fat Meat
    1 Bread
    2 Fat

Estimated nutrients per serving:

CAL	312	FAT	20
CHO	14	Na	983
PRO	19	K	432

Ingredients

  1 TABLESPOON MARGARINE
½ CUP CHOPPED ONION
  2 TABLESPOONS FLOUR
  2 CUPS BEEF BOUILLON
  2 TABLESPOONS SHERRY
  2 TABLESPOONS CATSUP
½ RECIPE OVEN MEATBALLS
¼ CUP DAIRY SOUR CREAM

Method

1. Melt margarine in frying pan. Add onion and cook until clear.
2. Stir in flour.
3. Add bouillon, sherry, and catsup. Simmer over low heat until mixture bubbles. Stir constantly.
4. Add Oven Meatballs. Cook until heated through.
5. Add sour cream and heat 1 or 2 minutes until sauce bubbles.

Serving suggestion: May be served over rice or noodles. Remember to add the Bread Exchanges. The sauce may be used with other meats.

Oven Meatballs in Spaghetti Sauce

Yield: 2 cups sauce (4 servings) Estimated nutrients per serving:
Exchanges per ½-cup sauce and
6-meatball serving:

	CAL	321	FAT 17
	CHO	20	Na 1147
	PRO	22	K 886

   2 Medium-Fat Meat
   1 Vegetable
   1 Bread
 1½ Fat

Ingredients

 ¼ CUP CHOPPED ONION
 ¼ CUP CHOPPED GREEN PEPPER
  1 TEASPOON VEGETABLE OIL
  1 16-OUNCE CAN TOMATOES
  1 8-OUNCE CAN TOMATO SAUCE
 ½ CUP MUSHROOM STEMS AND PIECES, DRAINED
 ½ TEASPOON CRUSHED OREGANO
 ½ TEASPOON CRUSHED BASIL
 ½ TEASPOON GARLIC SALT
  2 TEASPOONS BROWN SUGAR
 ½ RECIPE OVEN MEATBALLS
 ¼ CUP GRATED PARMESAN CHEESE

Method

1. In frying pan cook onion and green pepper in oil until tender.
2. Add tomatoes, tomato sauce, mushrooms, oregano, basil, garlic salt, and brown sugar. Mix well.
3. Add Oven Meatballs.
4. Simmer uncovered for 30 minutes, stirring occasionally.
5. Serve over hot, cooked spaghetti and sprinkle each serving with 1 tablespoon Parmesan cheese. Add Bread Exchanges for the spaghetti.

Meat Loaf

Yield: 6 servings
Exchanges per 1½-inch slice
serving:

3 Medium-Fat Meat
1 Vegetable
½ Bread
½ Fat

Estimated nutrients per serving:

CAL	335	FAT	19
CHO	16	Na	1040
PRO	25	K	653

Ingredients

1½ POUNDS GROUND BEEF
1 CUP FINE DRY BREAD CRUMBS
2 EGGS
1 8-OUNCE CAN TOMATO SAUCE
½ CUP CHOPPED ONION
2 TABLESPOONS CHOPPED GREEN PEPPER
1½ TEASPOONS SALT
1 MEDIUM BAY LEAF, CRUSHED
DASH THYME
DASH MARJORAM

Method

1. Preheat oven to 350° F.
2. Combine all ingredients; mix well.
3. Pat into 9-inch loaf pan.
4. Bake in oven for 1 hour.

Variation: For a smaller family, this recipe may be divided into 2
or 3 small loaves. One loaf can be used immediately and the others
frozen. Be sure to label each loaf with the number of servings and
exchanges per serving.
One-half of recipe or 2 loaves = 3-serving loaf
One-third of recipe or 3 loaves = 2-serving loaf

Meat Loaf Pie

Yield: 6 servings
Exchanges per 1-wedge serving:

    2 High-Fat Meat
    1 Vegetable
    1 Bread
    ½ Fat

Estimated nutrients per serving:

CAL	314	FAT	18
CHO	19	Na	1007
PRO	19	K	635

Ingredients

Meat Loaf

    1 POUND GROUND BEEF
    1 EGG
    1 SLICE BREAD, CUBED
    ¼ CUP MINCED ONION
    ⅔ CUP SKIM MILK
    2 TEASPOONS WORCESTERSHIRE SAUCE
    1 TEASPOON SALT

Potato Topping

    2 CUPS WATER
    ½ CUP SKIM MILK
    1 TABLESPOON MARGARINE
    ¾ TEASPOON SALT
    2 CUPS INSTANT MASHED POTATO FLAKES
    ¼ CUP SHREDDED CHEDDAR CHEESE (1 OUNCE)

Method

1. Heat oven to 350° F.
2. Mix all meat loaf ingredients in mixing bowl; pat out in 9-inch round cake pan.
3. Bake 45 minutes. Remove from oven, drain off excess fat.
4. While meat loaf is baking, make mashed potatoes. Put water, milk, margarine, and salt in saucepan. Bring to boil; remove from heat.

5. Stir in potato flakes with fork. Mix until fluffy. Keep warm on low heat.
6. Spread potatoes on meat loaf with a spatula. Sprinkle with cheese.
7. Return to oven until cheese melts (about 3 minutes).
8. Cut into 6 wedges and serve hot.

Beef Cheese Cups

Yield: 8 servings
Exchanges per 1-meat-cup serving:

1 Medium-Fat Meat
1 Vegetable
1 Fat

Estimated nutrients per serving:

CAL	154	FAT	10
CHO	4	Na	199
PRO	12	K	235

Ingredients

1 POUND GROUND BEEF
½ CUP CHEESE CRACKERS, CRUSHED
2 TABLESPOONS FINELY CHOPPED ONION
1 TABLESPOON FINELY CHOPPED GREEN PEPPER
2 TABLESPOONS CHILI SAUCE
2 DROPS TABASCO SAUCE
⅓ CUP SKIM MILK
1 EGG
¼ TEASPOON SALT
DASH PEPPER

Method

1. Preheat oven to 350° F.
2. Mix ingredients thoroughly in bowl.
3. Coat muffin pans with vegetable pan spray. Divide meat in 8 muffin wells.
4. Bake 40 minutes.

Beef Hash

Yield: 4 servings
Exchanges per 1-cup serving:
   ½ Milk
   2 Lean Meat
   ½ Bread

Estimated nutrients per serving:

CAL	195	FAT	7
CHO	14	Na	668
PRO	19	K	579

Ingredients

   2 CUPS LEAN COOKED BEEF, COARSELY GROUND
1½ CUPS COOKED, DICED POTATO
  ½ CUP CHOPPED ONION
  1 TEASPOON SALT
  ¼ TEASPOON PEPPER
  1 TEASPOON WORCESTERSHIRE SAUCE
  ½ CUP EVAPORATED SKIM MILK
  2 TABLESPOONS GRATED CHEDDAR CHEESE (ABOUT
    ½ OUNCE)

Method

1. Preheat oven to 350° F.
2. Lightly mix all ingredients except cheese in large frying pan.
3. Cook on low heat until underside is lightly browned.
4. Turn into 1½-quart casserole which has been sprayed with vegetable cooking spray. Top with cheese.
5. Heat in oven for 10 minutes to melt cheese.

Variation: ¾ pound raw ground beef, browned and drained, may be used in place of cooked beef. Exchanges are unchanged.

Curried Beef and Rice

Yield: 6 cups (6 servings)
Exchanges per 1-cup serving:
    2 Medium-Fat Meat
    1 Bread

Estimated nutrients per serving:

CAL	215	FAT	11
CHO	12	Na	375*
PRO	17	K	333

Ingredients

- 1 9-OUNCE PACKAGE FROZEN FRENCH-CUT GREEN BEANS
- 1 POUND GROUND BEEF
- ¾ CUP SLICED ONION
- ½ CUP UNCOOKED LONG GRAIN RICE
- 2 CUPS BEEF BROTH
- 1 4-OUNCE CAN MUSHROOM STEMS AND PIECES, DRAINED
- 1 TEASPOON CURRY POWDER
- 1 TEASPOON WORCESTERSHIRE SAUCE
- SALT TO TASTE*

Method

1. Cook green beans according to package instructions. Drain.
2. Brown beef in a large skillet. Drain.
3. Add remaining ingredients. Bring to boil over medium heat.
4. Cover, reduce heat; simmer until rice is done, about 15 or 20 minutes. Add extra water if too thick.
5. Stir in drained green beans.

Variation: Cold roast beef or other leftover cooked meat may be used in place of ground beef. Use 3 cups of diced meat for the same Exchanges.

*Na content of salt not included in estimate.

Beef Stroganoff Crepes

Yield: 12 crepes (6 servings)
Exchanges per 2-crepe serving:

    2 Medium-Fat Meat
    1 Bread
    1 Vegetable
    3 Fat

Estimated nutrients per serving:

CAL	385	FAT	25
CHO	20	Na	747
PRO	20	K	297

Ingredients

  ¼ CUP CHOPPED ONION
  1 POUND GROUND BEEF
  1 10½-OUNCE CAN CREAM OF MUSHROOM SOUP
  ½ TEASPOON SALT
  1 TABLESPOON CATSUP
  1 2-OUNCE CAN SLICED MUSHROOMS, DRAINED
  ½ CUP DAIRY SOUR CREAM
  12 PREPARED BASIC CREPES (SEE INDEX)
  1 TABLESPOON MELTED MARGARINE

Method

1. Preheat oven to 350° F.
2. In skillet sprayed with vegetable pan spray, saute onion and beef. Drain excess fat.
3. Add soup, salt, catsup, and mushrooms. Heat to boil. Remove from heat.
4. Stir in sour cream.
5. Put ¼ cup filling in center of each crepe; overlap sides. Place seam side down in 13-✕ 9-inch baking dish. Brush with melted margarine.
6. Heat for 10 to 15 minutes.

Baked Stuffed Cabbage

Yield: 8 rolls (4 servings)
Exchanges per 2-roll serving:
    3 Medium-Fat Meat
    1 Vegetable

Estimated nutrients per serving:

CAL	265	FAT	17
CHO	6	Na	692
PRO	22	K	628

Ingredients

  8 LARGE CABBAGE LEAVES
  1 POUND GROUND BEEF
  3 TABLESPOONS CHOPPED ONION
  2 TABLESPOONS CHOPPED PARSLEY
  ¾ TEASPOON SALT
  ½ TEASPOON THYME
  ½ CLOVE GARLIC, PRESSED
    DASH CAYENNE
  ½ CUP TOMATO SAUCE

Method

1. Preheat oven to 375° F.
2. Wash and blanch cabbage leaves. Drain and dry.
3. Combine remaining ingredients except tomato sauce. Divide meat mixture into 8 equal portions on cabbage leaves. Roll leaves around meat. Secure with toothpick.
4. Place seam side down in a casserole. Cover with tomato sauce.
5. Bake covered about 50 or 60 minutes.

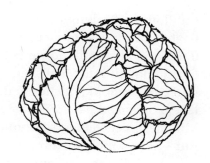

Beef Pasties

Yield: 6 pasties

Exchanges per 1-pasty serving:

    2 Medium-Fat Meat

    1 Vegetable

    2 Bread

    1 Fat

Estimated nutrients per serving:

CAL	357	FAT	17
CHO	34	Na	684
PRO	17	K	449

Ingredients

Crust

1½ CUPS FLOUR

 ¾ TEASPOON SALT

 ¼ CUP + 2 TEASPOONS VEGETABLE SHORTENING

 1 EGG

    WATER

Filling

 ¾ POUND COARSELY GROUND BEEF (RAW)

 2 CUPS DICED RAW POTATO

 ¾ CUP DICED CARROTS

 ¾ CUP CHOPPED ONION

 1 TEASPOON SALT

 ¼ TEASPOON PEPPER

 2 TABLESPOONS WATER

Method

1. Put flour and salt in mixing bowl. Cut in shortening.
2. Beat egg in measuring cup. Add water to make ½ cup. Add to flour, and mix until moistened.
3. Divide dough into 6 balls. On lightly floured board, roll balls into circles about 8 inches in diameter. Place circles between layers of waxed paper. Set aside.
4. Mix meat, vegetables, seasoning, and water.
5. Put 1 cup of meat mixture on each crust, placing it toward one side. Fold dough over and seal edges with fork tines. Pierce top with fork.

6. Place on baking sheet sprayed with vegetable pan spray.
7. Bake in 350° F oven for 45 minutes or until lightly browned.

Serving Suggestion: A pasty is a meal-in-a-crust, delicious and hearty. It needs only a crisp salad and fruit to complete the menu.

Layered Beef Vegetable Casserole

Yield: 8 cups (8 servings)
Exchanges per 1-cup serving:
    2 Medium-Fat Meat
    1 Vegetable
    1 Bread
    ½ Fat

Estimated nutrients per serving:

CAL	261	FAT	13
CHO	18	Na	816
PRO	18	K	720

Ingredients

1½ POUNDS GROUND BEEF
1 CUP SLICED ONION
1 CUP CHOPPED GREEN PEPPER
2 TEASPOONS SALT
1 LARGE POTATO, PEELED AND SLICED (½ POUND)
1 CUP THINLY SLICED CARROT
⅓ CUP LONG GRAIN RICE, UNCOOKED
1 28-OUNCE CAN TOMATOES, MASHED

Method

1. Preheat oven to 350° F.
2. Saute ground beef, onions, and green pepper together until beef is browned. Drain fat. Add salt; mix well.
3. Place sliced potato in bottom of 2½-quart baking dish.
4. Alternate layers of carrots, rice, and meat.
5. Pour mashed tomatoes over casserole. Cover.
6. Bake for 2 hours.

Taco Casserole

Yield: 4½ cups (9 servings)
Exchanges per ½-cup serving:
    2 Medium-Fat Meat
    ½ Vegetable
    1 Fat

Estimated nutrients per serving:

CAL	207	FAT	15
CHO	3	Na	397
PRO	15	K	188

Ingredients

   1 POUND GROUND BEEF
  ½ CUP CHOPPED ONION
   1 PACKAGE TACO SEASONING MIX (1¼ OUNCES)
1½ CUPS WATER
   1 CUP COARSELY CRUSHED TORTILLA CHIPS (ABOUT
     2 OUNCES)
1½ CUPS SHREDDED CHEDDAR CHEESE (ABOUT 6
     OUNCES)
  ½ CUP CHOPPED GREEN PEPPER

Method

1. Brown ground beef with onion in skillet. Drain.
2. Add seasoning mix and water to meat. Bring to a boil, reduce heat, and simmer 15 minutes.
3. Preheat oven to 350° F.
4. Spread corn chips on bottom of 8- × 8-inch baking dish. Pour meat sauce evenly over chips. Sprinkle cheese and green pepper over meat.
5. Bake in oven for 20 minutes or long enough to melt cheese and heat through.
6. Let stand 5 minutes before serving.

Tacos

Yield: 12 tacos (6 servings)
Exchanges per 2-taco serving:
    2 Medium-Fat Meat
    2 Bread
    1 Fat

Estimated nutrients per serving:

CAL	329	FAT	17
CHO	24	Na	445
PRO	20	K	458

Ingredients

  1 POUND GROUND BEEF
  1 PACKAGE TACO SEASONING MIX
  1 CUP WATER
12 TACO SHELLS

Toppings
1 CUP SHREDDED LETTUCE
1 CUP DICED TOMATOES
½ CUP CHOPPED ONION
½ CUP CHOPPED GREEN PEPPER
¾ CUP GRATED CHEDDAR CHEESE (3 OUNCES)

Method

1. Cook ground beef over medium heat in a skillet, stirring until brown and crumbly. Drain excess fat.
2. Add seasoning mix and water. Stir, bring to a boil. Reduce heat; simmer 10 minutes.
3. Warm taco shells in oven according to package directions.
4. To serve, place 3 tablespoons meat mixture in shell. Add vegetable toppings as desired and 1 tablespoon grated cheese.

Chile Con Carne

Yield: 6 cups (6 servings)
Exchanges per 1-cup serving:

 3 Lean Meat
 1 Vegetable
 2 Bread
 ½ Fat

Estimated nutrients per serving:

CAL	360	FAT	12
CHO	38	Na	717
PRO	25	K	1167

Ingredients

 1 POUND GROUND BEEF
 ½ CUP CHOPPED ONION
 ½ CUP CHOPPED GREEN PEPPER
 2 1-POUND CANS KIDNEY BEANS
 2 CUPS CANNED TOMATOES
 1 8-OUNCE CAN TOMATO SAUCE
 2 TEASPOONS CHILI POWDER
 1 TEASPOON SALT
 1 BAY LEAF
    DASH PAPRIKA
    DASH CAYENNE

Method

1. Brown meat with onion and green pepper. Drain off excess fat.
2. Add remaining ingredients.
3. Cover and simmer 1 hour, adding extra water if needed.

Lima Bean-Meatball Casserole

Yield: 8 cups (8 servings)
Exchanges per 1-cup serving:

2 Lean Meat
1 Vegetable
1 Bread
½ Fat

Estimated nutrients per serving:

CAL	241	FAT	9
CHO	24	Na	392
PRO	16	K	707

Ingredients

1 CUP DRIED LIMA BEANS
5 CUPS WATER, DIVIDED
¼ CUP FLOUR
1 CUP CANNED TOMATOES
1 CUP SLICED CELERY
1 CUP SLICED CARROT
½ CUP CHOPPED ONION
1 BAY LEAF
1 TEASPOON SALT
¼ CUP DRY BREAD CRUMBS
¼ CUP SKIM MILK
¼ TEASPOON WORCESTERSHIRE SAUCE
1 POUND GROUND BEEF

Method

1. Place beans in Dutch oven with 4½ cups water. Boil 2 minutes; cover; remove from heat; let stand 1 hour.
2. Combine flour and ½ cup water. Stir into beans. Cook until thickened.
3. Add vegetables, bay leaf, and salt. Cover; bake at 375° F for 1 hour.
4. Make 16 small meatballs with remaining ingredients. Add to stew; continue baking 45 minutes.

Lentils with Franks

Yield: 4 cups (4 servings)
Exchanges per 1-cup serving:

    2 High-Fat Meat

    2 Bread

    ½ Fat

Estimated nutrients per serving:

CAL	362	FAT	18
CHO	31	Na	907
PRO	19	K	511

Ingredients

  1 CUP RAW LENTILS
2½ CUPS WATER
  1 BAY LEAF
  ½ TEASPOON SALT
  ¼ CUP CHOPPED ONION
  ½ POUND FRANKFURTERS, CUT IN ½-INCH SLICES

Method

1. Wash lentils. Place in heavy saucepan with water, bay leaf, and salt. Simmer 35 minutes or until tender.
2. While lentils simmer, brown onions and frankfurters in skillet sprayed with vegetable pan spray.
3. Drain lentils; remove bay leaf.
4. Add frankfurters and onions.

Variation: Substitute chicken or beef stock for water.

Broiled Liver

Yield: 4 servings
Exchanges per 1-slice serving:
    2 Lean Meat
    1 Vegetable
    ½ Fat

Estimated nutrients per serving:
CAL	173	FAT	9
CHO	6	Na	321
PRO	17	K	251

Ingredients

  ¾ POUND BEEF LIVER (ABOUT 4 SLICES)
  ¼ CUP FRENCH DRESSING

Method

1. Remove membrane from liver. Snip out veins with kitchen shears. Cut into 4 portions if necessary.
2. Brush slices of liver with French dressing.
3. Broil 3 inches from heat for 3 minutes. Turn and broil 3 or 4 minutes longer.

Serving suggestion: Serve with pan-fried onions (see recipe).

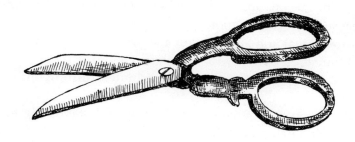

Shish Kabob

Yield: 4 servings
Exchanges per 1 skewer serving:

    3 Lean Meat

    2 Vegetable

    ½ Fat

Estimated nutrients per serving:

CAL	248	FAT	12
CHO	11	Na	354
PRO	24	K	1015

Ingredients

  1 POUND BEEF SIRLOIN
  ½ CUP VINEGAR
  2 TABLESPOONS SALAD OIL
  1 MEDIUM ONION, CHOPPED
  2 TABLESPOONS CHOPPED FRESH PARSLEY
  ½ TEASPOON SALT
  ⅛ TEASPOON PEPPER
  1 GREEN PEPPER, CUT IN WIDE STRIPS
  6 SMALL TOMATOES, HALVED

Method

1. Trim fat from meat. Cut meat into 1½-inch cubes.
2. Mix vinegar, oil, onion, parsley, salt, and pepper. Marinate meat in mixture for 2 hours, stirring occasionally.
3. Remove meat and alternate on 4 skewers with green pepper and tomatoes. Brush with marinade.
4. Broil 4 inches from heat about 10 minutes, turning once.

Variation: If you do not have skewers, the shish kabob ingredients may be broiled in a pan. Follow steps 1 and 2 above. Then arrange meat, pepper, and tomato separately in pan. Sprinkle 1 teaspoon of marinating mixture on vegetables; broil until tender, stirring once. Arrange on platter for serving.

Savory Lamb Stew

Yield: 6 scant cups
Exchanges per 1-cup serving:

    3 Lean Meat
    1 Vegetable
    2 Bread
    1 Fat

Estimated nutrients per serving:

CAL	361	FAT	13
CHO	35	Na	899
PRO	26	K	1143

Ingredients

  ¼ CUP FLOUR
  2 POUNDS LEAN LAMB, CUT IN 1½-INCH CUBES
  2 TABLESPOONS VEGETABLE OIL
  ¾ CUP BEEF BROTH
1½ TEASPOONS SALT
  1 TEASPOON CRUMBLED LEAF THYME
  ¼ TEASPOON PEPPER
  6 SMALL NEW POTATOES, PARED
  6 CARROTS, CUT IN 1-INCH PIECES
  1 28-OUNCE CAN TOMATOES, DRAINED

Method
1. Shake flour with meat in plastic bag to coat.
2. Heat oil in heavy kettle. Brown meat.
3. Stir in broth, salt, thyme, and pepper.
4. Cover and simmer 45 minutes.
5. Add potatoes and carrots. Cover and simmer 45 minutes or until vegetables are done.
6. Add tomatoes and heat.

Curried Lamb on Rice

Yield: 3 cups (4 servings)
Exchanges per ¾-cup meat over
½-cup rice serving:

2 Lean Meat
½ Vegetable
2 Bread
½ Fat

Estimated nutrients per serving:

CAL	285	FAT	9
CHO	32	NA	995
PRO	19	K	406

Ingredients

    1 POUND LEAN LAMB, CUBED, TRIMMED OF FAT
    ½ CUP CHOPPED ONION
    1 CLOVE GARLIC, MINCED (OPTIONAL)
    1 TABLESPOON MARGARINE
    2 TEASPOONS CURRY POWDER
    ¾ TEASPOON SALT
    ¼ TEASPOON GROUND GINGER
    1 MEDIUM TOMATO, PEELED AND CHOPPED
 1½ TABLESPOONS FLOUR
    1 CUBE BEEF BOUILLON
    1 CUP BOILING WATER
    ½ CUP GRATED CARROT
    2 CUPS COOKED RICE

Method

1. Brown lamb, onion, and garlic in margarine.
2. Add curry powder, salt, ginger, tomato, and flour. Mix well. Dissolve bouillon cube in water; stir into meat.
3. Cover and simmer 30 to 40 minutes or until lamb is tender. Stir occasionally.
4. Toss rice with grated carrot.
5. Serve lamb over rice.

Veal Parmesan

Yield: 4 servings
Exchanges per serving (1 piece
veal with ¼ cup sauce):
    4 Medium-Fat Meat
    1 Vegetable
    ½ Bread

Estimated nutrients per serving:

CAL	371	FAT	23
CHO	11	Na	1095*
PRO	30	K	757

Ingredients

  3 TABLESPOONS MARGARINE
  ½ CUP CORN FLAKE CRUMBS
  3 TABLESPOONS PARMESAN CHEESE
  ½ TEASPOON SALT
    DASH PEPPER
  1 POUND VEAL CUTLETS, ¼ INCH THICK
  1 EGG, BEATEN
  1 8-OUNCE CAN TOMATO SAUCE
  ¼ TEASPOON OREGANO
    DASH ONION SALT*
  2 OUNCES MOZZARELLA CHEESE

Method

1. Preheat oven to 400° F.
2. Melt margarine in 10- × 6-inch baking dish.
3. Combine crumbs, Parmesan cheese, salt, and pepper.
4. Cut veal into 4 serving pieces. Dip in egg, then in crumbs. Place in baking dish.
5. Bake for 20 minutes. Turn meat and bake 15 to 20 minutes more or until tender.
6. In saucepan combine remaining ingredients except cheese. Bring to boil. Pour over meat.
7. Divide cheese into 4 portions. Place one on each piece of veal.
8. Return to oven to melt cheese.

*Na content of onion salt not included in estimate.

Veal Paprika

Yield: 6 servings

Exchanges per 1/6-recipe serving:

   3 Lean Meat

   ½ Bread

   3 Fat

Estimated nutrients per serving:

CAL	322	FAT	22
CHO	7	Na	541
PRO	24	K	528

Ingredients

- 1½ POUNDS VEAL STEAK OR CUTLETS, ½ INCH THICK
- ¼ CUP FLOUR
- 1 TEASPOON SALT
- ¼ TEASPOON PEPPER
- ½ CUP SLICED ONION
- 1 CLOVE GARLIC, MINCED
- 2 TABLESPOONS VEGETABLE OIL
- ⅓ CUP BEEF CONSOMME, CONDENSED
- 1 TABLESPOON PAPRIKA
- 3 DROPS TABASCO SAUCE
- 1 CUP DAIRY SOUR CREAM

Method

1. Cut meat into 6 pieces. Pound until double in size.
2. Combine flour, salt, and pepper. Dredge veal in flour mixture.
3. Saute onion and garlic in oil until tender. Remove from pan. Add meat to oil and brown.
4. Add onion, garlic, and remaining ingredients except sour cream. Simmer, covered, 15 minutes or until meat is tender.
5. Stir in sour cream. Heat through.

Oriental Veal and Sprouts

Yield: 6 servings

Exchanges per serving (⅓ cup veal on ⅓ cup bean sprouts):

   3 Medium-Fat Meat
   1 Vegetable

Estimated nutrients per serving:

CAL	260	FAT	16
CHO	5	Na	506
PRO	24	K	517

Ingredients

1½ POUNDS VEAL, CUT INTO THIN STRIPS
  3 TABLESPOONS VEGETABLE OIL, DIVIDED
  3 GREEN ONIONS, SLICED
  1 GARLIC CLOVE, CRUSHED
  1 TABLESPOON FLOUR
  2 TABLESPOONS SOY SAUCE
  1 16-OUNCE CAN BEAN SPROUTS, DRAINED

Method

1. Brown veal strips in 2 tablespoons hot oil.
2. Add onions and garlic; saute about 5 minutes, stirring constantly.
3. Sprinkle flour over mixture, stirring until blended.
4. Add soy sauce. Cover and cook about 15 minutes or until veal is tender.
5. While meat cooks, stir-fry bean sprouts lightly in 1 tablespoon oil until heated.
6. Serve meat with sauce on bed of sprouts.

Hawaiian Pork Chops

Yield: 6 chops with sauce
Exchanges per 1-chop serving:

    2 Lean Meat
    1 Vegetable
    1 Fruit

Estimated nutrients per serving:

CAL	179	FAT	7
CHO	15	Na	502
PRO	14	K	340

Ingredients

- ½ CUP CHOPPED ONION
- ½ CUP CHOPPED GREEN PEPPER
- 2 TABLESPOONS FLOUR
- 1 TEASPOON SALT
- ¼ TEASPOON PEPPER
- 6 LOIN PORK CHOPS, TRIMMED (EACH ABOUT 4 OUNCES WITH BONE)
- 6 PINEAPPLE SLICES, UNSWEETENED (DRAIN JUICE AND RESERVE)
- 1 TABLESPOON VINEGAR
- ¼ CUP CATSUP
- ½ CUP PINEAPPLE JUICE

Method

1. In large skillet sprayed with vegetable pan spray, cook onion and green pepper until onion is clear. Remove from skillet.
2. Mix flour, salt, and pepper in plastic bag. Add chops, one at a time; shake to coat meat.
3. Brown chops in skillet.
4. Place pineapple slice on top of each chop. Sprinkle with onion and green pepper.
5. Combine vinegar, catsup, and juice to make sauce. Pour over chops. Simmer 45 minutes or until chops are done.

Pork Chow Mein

Yield: 6 cups
Exchanges per 1-cup serving:
    2 Medium-Fat Meat
    2 Vegetable

Estimated nutrients per serving:

CAL	214	FAT	10
CHO	12	Na	1156
PRO	19	K	626

Ingredients

  1 POUND PORK, CUT IN THIN STRIPS
  1 TABLESPOON VEGETABLE OIL, DIVIDED
  3 CUPS SLICED CELERY, BIAS CUT
  1 CUP SLICED ONIONS
  2 4-OUNCE CANS MUSHROOMS, SLICED
2½ TABLESPOONS CORNSTARCH
10 OUNCES BEEF BROTH
¼ CUP SOY SAUCE
  1 1-POUND CAN BEAN SPROUTS, DRAINED

Method

1. Brown pork in 1 teaspoon oil. Drain.
2. Cook celery, onions, and mushrooms in 2 teaspoons oil until tender crisp, 2 or 3 minutes, stirring often. Drain excess fat.
3. Stir cornstarch into broth.
4. Combine all ingredients. Mix well.
5. Heat, stirring, until liquid is thickened and pork is completely cooked.

Serving suggestions: Pork Chow Mein may be served over one of the following:
½ cup cooked rice = 1 Bread Exchange
½ cup chow mein noodles = 1 Bread, 1 Fat Exchange

Sauerkraut and Pork Chops

Yield: 4 servings

Exchanges per serving (1 pork chop with ½ cup sauerkraut):

2 Lean Meat
1 Vegetable
½ Fruit

Estimated nutrients per serving:

CAL	151	FAT	7
CHO	8	Na	905
PRO	14	K	361

Ingredients

4 LEAN LOIN PORK CHOPS (1 POUND)
2 CUPS SAUERKRAUT, DRAINED (ABOUT 1 POUND)
1 SMALL APPLE, PEELED AND SLICED
1 TEASPOON CARAWAY SEEDS (OPTIONAL)

Method

1. Brown pork chops in skillet. Mix sauerkraut with meat juices in skillet.
2. Layer half of sauerkraut, half of apple slices, and half of caraway seeds in casserole.
3. Arrange pork chops over top of mixture.
4. Layer remaining sauerkraut, apple, and caraway seeds.
5. Cover and bake in 350° F oven for 1½ hours or until pork is tender.

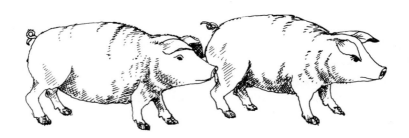

Baked Spareribs with Barbecue Sauce

Yield: 6 servings

Exchanges per 1/6-recipe serving:
    2 High-Fat Meat
    1 Vegetable
    1 Fat

Estimated nutrients per serving:

CAL	279	FAT	23
CHO	4	Na	720
PRO	14	K	476

Ingredients

  2 POUNDS PORK SPARERIBS, LEAN
  1 GARLIC CLOVE, MINCED
  3 TABLESPOONS VINEGAR
  1 8-OUNCE CAN TOMATO SAUCE
  ⅓ CUP CHOPPED ONION
1½ TEASPOONS CHILI POWDER
  1 TEASPOON SALT
  ¼ TEASPOON PEPPER
  ½ TEASPOON OREGANO
  ½ CUP WATER

Method

1. Trim excess fat from ribs. Cut into 6 serving portions. Place in baking pan.
2. Combine remaining ingredients; pour over ribs. Cover and let stand 15 minutes.
3. Preheat oven to 350° F.
4. Bake covered for 1½ hours.
5. Remove cover; baste; bake ½ hour.
6. Spoon off excess fat before serving.

Beef Macaroni Skillet Dinner

Yield: 6 servings

Exchanges per 1-cup serving:

    2 Medium-Fat Meat

    1 Vegetable

    1 Bread

    1 Fat

Estimated nutrients per serving:

CAL	299	FAT	15
CHO	21	Na	NA
PRO	20	K	NA

Ingredients

    1 CUP UNCOOKED MACARONI

    1 8-OUNCE CAN TOMATO SAUCE

    1 POUND GROUND BEEF

    ½ CUP GRATED CHEDDAR CHEESE (ABOUT 2 OUNCES)

    ⅓ CUP WHOLE KERNEL CORN, CANNED OR FROZEN

    1 TABLESPOON DEHYDRATED MINCED ONION

    2 CUPS CUT GREEN BEANS, CANNED OR FROZEN

    ¼ TEASPOON SALT

    1 TABLESPOON WORCESTERSHIRE SAUCE

    DASH BASIL (OPTIONAL)

    ¼ CUP WATER

Method

1. Cook macaroni according to package directions. Drain; add tomato sauce.
2. Brown beef in large skillet. Drain well.
3. Add macaroni to skillet; add remaining ingredients. Mix; cover and simmer over low heat until bubbly.
4. Add more water if mixture becomes dry.

Chunky Bar-B-Q Beef

Yield: 8 servings
Exchanges per ⅔-cup serving:

   3 Lean Meat
   ½ Vegetable
   ½ Bread
   ½ Fat

Estimated nutrients per serving:

CAL	232	FAT	12
CHO	10	Na	NA
PRO	21	K	NA

Ingredients

1¾ POUNDS LEAN BEEF, CUT IN SMALL CUBES
  1 1½-OUNCE PACKAGE DRY ONION SOUP MIX
2½ CUPS TOMATO JUICE
 ½ CUP WATER
 ½ CUP CATSUP
   SALT AND PEPPER TO TASTE

Method

1. Preheat oven to 325° F.
2. Brown meat in large skillet sprayed with vegetable pan spray.
3. Add remaining ingredients. Mix; place in a 2-quart casserole. Cover.
4. Bake for 2 hours. More water may be added if desired.

Serving suggestion: Serve over rice, noodles, or potatoes: ½ cup adds one Bread Exchange.

Main Dishes: Poultry

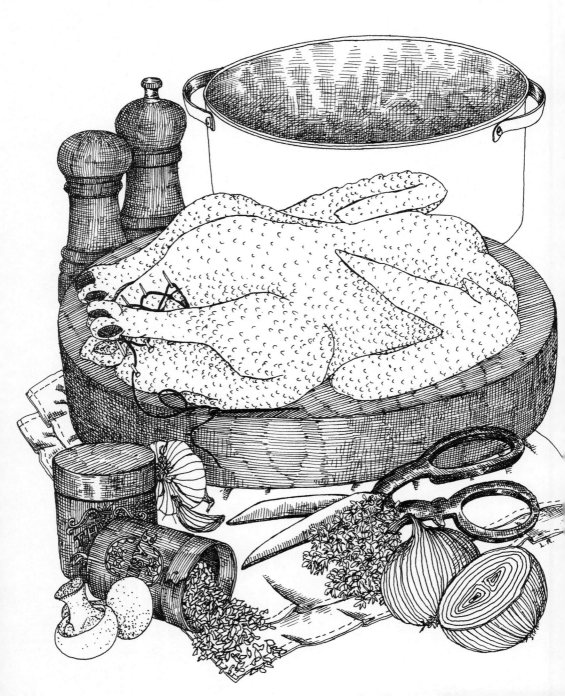

Chicken and turkey may be prepared in many ways. In addition to the recipes in this section, remember to try the chicken salads.

Poultry has the additional advantage of being in the low-fat meat category. You will note that the skin is removed from the chicken in these recipes.

Chicken and turkey leftovers have so many uses that they are a joy to the menu planner. Try the recipes in this section for a change from turkey sandwiches.

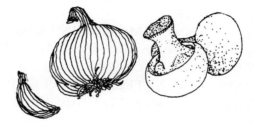

Chicken with Wine Sauce

Yield: 4 servings

Exchanges per serving (½ breast with sauce, ½ cup rice):

    4 Lean Meat
    2 Bread

Estimated nutrients per serving:

CAL	346	FAT	10
CHO	34	Na	636
PRO	30	K	370

Ingredients

- 1½ TABLESPOONS FLOUR
- ½ TEASPOON SALT
- ⅛ TEASPOON PEPPER
- 2 CHICKEN BREASTS, SPLIT, BONED, AND SKINNED (4 HALVES)
- 2 TABLESPOONS MARGARINE, DIVIDED
- 2 4-OUNCE CANS MUSHROOMS, THINLY SLICED
- ¼ CUP CHOPPED ONION
- 2 TABLESPOONS FRESH CHOPPED PARSLEY, DIVIDED
- 2 TABLESPOONS CORNSTARCH
- 1 CUP WATER
- ½ CUP WHITE WINE
- 1 CUBE CHICKEN BOUILLON
- 2 CUPS HOT COOKED RICE

Method

1. Combine flour, salt, and pepper in a plastic bag. Add 1 chicken piece at a time; shake to coat. Shake off excess.
2. Melt 1 tablespoon margarine in skillet over medium heat. Brown chicken, remove from skillet.
3. Add 1 tablespoon of margarine to skillet; saute mushrooms, onion, and 1 tablespoon parsley. Cook until onion is transparent. Remove from heat.

Home ↓

433-8494 oc

433-1000 oc

Cd Dry Crk Winery ↑

Larry at

4. Blend cornstarch and water. Add to mushroom onion mixture with wine and bouillon cube. Bring to a boil, stirring frequently.
5. When sauce starts to thicken, add chicken. Cover, reduce heat, and simmer 25 minutes or until chicken is tender, stirring occasionally. Add water if needed.
6. Serve with rice. Garnish with remaining parsley.

Parmesan Chicken Bake

Yield: 6 servings
Exchanges per 1-piece serving:
    4 Lean Meat

Estimated nutrients per serving:

CAL	219	FAT	11
CHO	3	Na	553
PRO	27	K	352

Ingredients

¼ CUP DRY BREAD CRUMBS
2 TABLESPOONS GRATED PARMESAN CHEESE
1 TABLESPOON PARSLEY FLAKES
1 TEASPOON SALT
⅛ TEASPOON LEMON PEPPER
⅛ TEASPOON THYME
3 CHICKEN BREASTS, SPLIT AND SKINNED (6 HALVES)
3 TABLESPOONS MELTED MARGARINE

Method

1. Preheat oven to 350° F.
2. Combine bread crumbs, cheese, and seasonings in shallow dish.
3. Dip chicken in crumb mixture. Coat both sides.
4. Melt margarine in baking dish in oven.
5. Add chicken, turning to coat both sides with margarine.
6. Bake, uncovered, for 1 hour.

Sesame Chicken Breasts

Yield: 6 pieces
Exchanges per 1-piece serving:

Estimated nutrients per serving:

4 Lean Meat	CAL	276	FAT 16
1 Vegetable	CHO	5	Na 235
1 Fat	PRO	28	K 360

Ingredients

- ¼ CUP FLOUR
- ½ TEASPOON SALT
- DASH PEPPER
- 3 CHICKEN BREASTS, SPLIT AND SKINNED (6 HALVES)
- 4 TABLESPOONS VEGETABLE OIL
- 4 TABLESPOONS SESAME SEEDS
- ½ CUP DRY WHITE WINE

Method

1. Preheat oven to 350° F.
2. Mix flour, salt, and pepper. Dip chicken in flour mixture. Coat on both sides.
3. Heat oil in baking pan in oven. Add chicken, turning to coat both sides with oil.
4. Sprinkle with half of sesame seeds.
5. Bake for 30 minutes. Turn chicken; sprinkle with remaining sesame seeds.
6. Pour wine into pan. Bake for 40 to 50 minutes more, until tender, basting occasionally.

California Chicken

Yield: 4 servings
Exchanges per 1-piece serving:
    4 Lean Meat
    ½ Bread
    ½ Fat
    1 Fruit

Estimated nutrients per serving:

CAL	322	FAT	14
CHO	21	Na	2237
PRO	28	K	527

Ingredients

  ⅓ CUP FLOUR
  ½ TEASPOON SALT
  ¼ TEASPOON CELERY SALT
  ¼ TEASPOON GROUND NUTMEG
  2 CHICKEN BREASTS, SPLIT AND SKINNED (4 HALVES)
  3 TABLESPOONS MARGARINE
  1 CUP PINEAPPLE JUICE
  ⅓ CUP SOY SAUCE
  1 TABLESPOON SUGAR

Method

1. Preheat oven to 350° F.
2. Mix dry ingredients. Dredge chicken in mixture.
3. Brown chicken in margarine in skillet.
4. Place in baking dish.
5. Combine remaining ingredients. Pour over chicken.
6. Bake, uncovered, for 1 hour. Baste every 15 minutes.

Chinese Ginger Chicken

Yield: 6 cups

Exchanges per 1-cup serving:

    2½ Lean Meat

    1 Vegetable

    ½ Bread

Estimated nutrients per serving:

CAL	167	FAT	3
CHO	14	Na	1204
PRO	21	K	533

Ingredients

⅓ CUP SOY SAUCE

2 TEASPOONS GINGER

2 WHOLE CHICKEN BREASTS, BONED AND SKINNED, CUT IN ¼-INCH STRIPS

1 16-OUNCE CAN BEAN SPROUTS

2 TABLESPOONS CORNSTARCH

½ CUP GREEN ONIONS, SLICED IN ¼-INCH PIECES

1 4-OUNCE CAN MUSHROOM SLICES, DRAINED

1 6-OUNCE CAN BAMBOO SHOOTS, DRAINED AND SLICED

1 9-OUNCE PACKAGE FROZEN CUT GREEN BEANS

1 CUP WATER

Method

1. Mix soy sauce and ginger.
2. Spray large skillet with vegetable pan spray. Add chicken and sauce. Cook on high heat for approximately 4 minutes. Remove chicken.
3. Drain bean sprouts, reserving liquid.
4. Cook bean sprout liquid with cornstarch in skillet, stirring until thickened. Add vegetables, chicken, and water.
5. Simmer until beans are tender-crisp and chicken is done.

Serving suggestions: Serve over cooked rice (add 1 Bread Exchange per ½ cup rice) or Chinese noodles (add 1 Bread and 1 Fat Exchange per ½-cup serving).

Chicken Subgum

Yield: 5 cups
Exchanges per 1-cup serving:
  2 Lean Meat
  1 Vegetable
  ½ Bread

Estimated nutrients per serving:
CAL 160   FAT   4
CHO 15   Na   1633
PRO 16   K   568

Ingredients

  2 CHICKEN BOUILLON CUBES
1½ CUPS WATER
  2 CUPS DICED COOKED CHICKEN (8 OUNCES)
1¼ CUPS SLICED CELERY
  1 16-OUNCE CAN CHINESE VEGETABLES, DRAINED
  1 8-OUNCE CAN WATER CHESTNUTS, DRAINED AND
    SLICED
1½ TEASPOONS DEHYDRATED MINCED ONION
  2 TABLESPOONS CORNSTARCH
  3 TABLESPOONS SOY SAUCE

Method

1. Dissolve bouillon cubes in hot water in saucepan.
2. Add remaining ingredients except cornstarch and soy sauce.
3. Heat to boiling. Reduce heat and simmer 10 minutes uncovered.
4. Mix cornstarch and soy sauce. Add to chicken mixture. Cook
   over medium heat, stirring constantly until thickened and clear.

Serving suggestion: May be served over chow mein noodles.
Add 1 Bread and 1 Fat Exchange for ½ cup noodles.

Chicken à la King

Yield: 6 cups

Exchanges per ¾-cup serving:

    4 Lean Meat

    ½ Bread

Estimated nutrients per serving:

CAL	247	FAT	11
CHO	8	Na	832
PRO	29	K	421

Ingredients

    2 CHICKEN BOUILLON CUBES
1½ CUPS HOT WATER
    3 TABLESPOONS MARGARINE
    3 TABLESPOONS FLOUR
2½ CUPS DICED COOKED CHICKEN
    1 CUP COOKED PEAS
    1 4-OUNCE CAN SLICED MUSHROOMS, DRAINED
    ½ CUP SLICED COOKED CARROTS
    ¼ CUP CHOPPED ONION
    2 TABLESPOONS CHOPPED PIMIENTO
    1 TEASPOON SALT

Method

1. Dissolve bouillon cubes in hot water.
2. In saucepan, melt margarine; blend in flour. Add broth slowly, stirring. Cook on medium heat until thick, stirring constantly.
3. Add other ingredients and heat until mixture bubbles.
4. Serve over biscuits, rice, toast, or other favorite. Remember to add the necessary Bread Exchange.

Turkey Broccoli Casserole

Yield: 6 servings

Exchanges per 1/6-recipe
serving:

   ½ Milk
   2 Medium-Fat Meat
   1 Vegetable

Estimated nutrients per serving:

CAL	206	FAT	10
CHO	9	Na	553
PRO	20	K	418

Ingredients

   2 10-OUNCE PACKAGES FROZEN BROCCOLI SPEARS
   2 CUPS COARSELY DICED COOKED TURKEY
   1 10½-OUNCE CAN CREAM OF MUSHROOM SOUP
  ½ CUP SKIM MILK
  ½ CUP GRATED CHEDDAR CHEESE (ABOUT 2 OUNCES)

Method

1. Preheat oven to 375° F.
2. Cook broccoli according to package directions. Layer in 12- × 8-inch baking dish.
3. Spread turkey evenly on top.
4. Combine soup with milk; mix until smooth and pour over turkey.
5. Sprinkle grated cheese on top.
6. Bake for 30 minutes. Let stand 5 minutes before cutting into 6 portions.

Turkey Pot Pie

Yield: 5 servings
Exchanges per 1-cup serving:
    2 Lean Meat
    2 Vegetable
    1 Bread
    2 Fat

Estimated nutrients per serving:

CAL	338	FAT	18
CHO	23	Na	693
PRO	21	K	256

Ingredients

- 2 CUPS DICED COOKED TURKEY
- 1 TABLESPOON FLOUR
- 1 CUP CHOPPED ONION
- ¼ CUP SLICED CELERY
- ½ TEASPOON CRUSHED THYME
- ⅛ TEASPOON PEPPER
- 1 TABLESPOON MARGARINE
- 1 CUP SLICED COOKED CARROTS
- ½ CUP WATER
- 1 10½-OUNCE CAN MUSHROOM SOUP
- 1 CUP COOKED CUT GREEN BEANS
- 1 PACKAGE READY-TO-BAKE REFRIGERATED BISCUITS (5 IN A PACKAGE)

Method

1. Preheat oven to 350° F.
2. Toss turkey with flour in plastic bag. Set aside.
3. In frying pan, cook onions and celery with thyme and pepper in margarine until tender.
4. Add carrots, water, soup, green beans, and turkey. Pour into 2-quart casserole.
5. Split biscuits in half and place on top. Bake for 30 minutes.

Chicken Cacciatore

Yield: 5 cups (4 servings)
Exchanges per 1¼-cup serving:

   3 Lean Meat
   1 Vegetable
  ½ Bread

Estimated nutrients per serving:

CAL	245	FAT	5
CHO	13	Na	NA
PRO	27	K	NA

Ingredients

   3 POUNDS FRYING CHICKEN, CUT UP
  ½ CUP CHOPPED ONION
  ¼ CUP CHOPPED GREEN PEPPER
  ½ CUP CHOPPED CELERY
   1 28-OUNCE CAN TOMATOES
  ½ TEASPOON SALT
   1 CLOVE GARLIC, MINCED
   1 TEASPOON PARSLEY FLAKES
    DASH OREGANO
   1 TABLESPOON CORNSTARCH
  ¼ CUP WATER

Method

1. Brown pieces of chicken in skillet sprayed with vegetable pan spray.
2. Add vegetables, salt, and spices. Cover and simmer 1 hour.
3. Mix cornstarch with water and add to skillet, stirring until gravy thickens.

Main Dishes:
Fish and Seafood

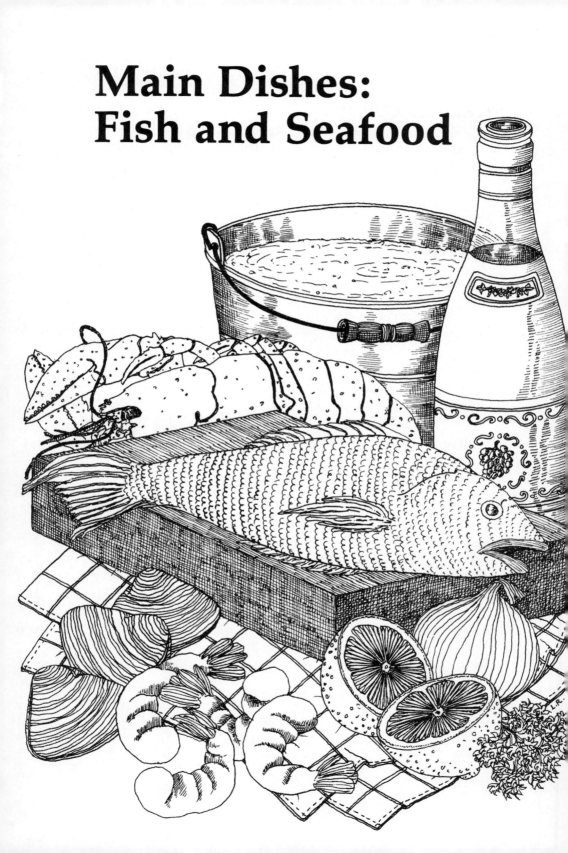

We are all being encouraged to eat more fish for its good nutrition and low fat content. It can be cooked in many ways, is quick to prepare, and is frequently an economical main dish. The choices here range from tuna dishes to elegant seafood.

Fish Baked in Foil

Yield: 4 servings

Exchanges per 3-ounce (approx.) serving:

   3 Lean Meat

Estimated nutrients per serving:

CAL	140	FAT	4
CHO	2	Na	160*
PRO	24	K	365

Ingredients

  4 FISH FILLETS—COD, PERCH, WHITEFISH, ETC. (1 POUND)
  1 TABLESPOON VEGETABLE OIL
    SALT* AND PEPPER TO TASTE
  1 SMALL CARROT, SLICED LENGTHWISE
  ½ MEDIUM ONION, SLICED
  1 TABLESPOON MINCED FRESH PARSLEY

Method

1. Preheat oven to 450° F.
2. Divide fish into 4 serving portions if necessary. Place each portion in center of a 12-inch square of foil.
3. Brush with oil. Sprinkle with salt and pepper.
4. Put carrot and onion on fish. Seal foil.
5. Place on shallow pan. Bake for 25 to 30 minutes.
6. Fold back foil, sprinkle fish with parsley. Serve in foil.

*Na content of salt not included in estimate.

Oven-Fried Fish

Yield: 4 servings

Exchanges per 3-ounce (approx.) serving:

    3 Lean Meat
    1 Bread

Estimated nutrients per serving:

CAL	197	FAT	5
CHO	12	Na	787
PRO	26	K	431

Ingredients

    4 FISH FILLETS (1 POUND)
    2 CUPS CORN FLAKES
    1 TEASPOON SALT
    ⅛ TEASPOON PEPPER
    ¼ CUP EVAPORATED SKIM MILK
    4 TEASPOONS VEGETABLE OIL

Method

1. Preheat oven to 500° F.
2. Cut fish into 4 serving pieces if necessary.
3. Roll corn flakes into fine crumbs between layers of waxed paper. Add salt and pepper.
4. Pour milk into shallow pan. Dip fish in milk, then in crumbs.
5. Arrange fish on baking sheet sprayed with vegetable pan spray.
6. Sprinkle oil over fish.
7. Bake for 10 minutes.

Tomatoed Fish Fillets

Yield: 4 fillets

Exchanges per 1-fillet serving:

    3 Lean Meat

    1 Vegetable

Estimated nutrients per serving:

CAL	157	FAT	5
CHO	4	Na	684
PRO	24	K	566

Ingredients

  1 POUND FROZEN COD FILLETS

¼ TEASPOON THYME

½ 10½-OUNCE CAN CREAM OF MUSHROOM SOUP

  1 MEDIUM TOMATO, SLICED

  1 TEASPOON MARGARINE

    DILL WEED AS DESIRED

Method

1. Preheat oven to 350° F.
2. Divide fillets into 4 serving portions. Place in ungreased baking dish.
3. Stir thyme into soup; spoon over fish. Bake uncovered for 30 minutes. Remove from oven.
4. Put 1 slice tomato on each fillet. Brush tomato with margarine; sprinkle with dill weed.
5. Bake 5 minutes longer or until fish flakes easily with fork.

Poached Fish Fillets

Yield: 4 servings

Exchanges per 3-ounce (approx.) serving:

3 Lean Meat*

Estimated nutrients per serving:

CAL	105	FAT	1
CHO	1	Na	639
PRO	23	K	350

Ingredients

    4 COD FILLETS (1 POUND)
2–3 CUPS WATER
    BAY LEAVES AS DESIRED
    PEPPERCORNS AS DESIRED
    1 TEASPOON SALT
    FRESH PARSLEY AS DESIRED
   ½ MEDIUM ONION, SLICED
    LEMON SLICES AS DESIRED

Method

1. Cut fish into 4 serving pieces if necessary.
2. Put all ingredients except fish in skillet. Simmer for 5 minutes.
3. Add fish; simmer gently 4 to 6 minutes or until fish flakes with fork. Do not overcook.

*Add one Fat Exchange to meal allowance.

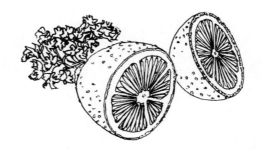

Tuna Loaf

Yield: 4 slices
Exchanges per 1-slice serving:
    4 Lean Meat
    ½ Bread

Estimated nutrients per serving:

CAL	268	FAT	12
CHO	8	Na	980*
PRO	32	K	422

Ingredients

- 2 6½-OUNCE CANS TUNA (IN WATER)
- 2 EGGS
- ¼ CUP CHOPPED ONION
- ¼ CUP CHOPPED WALNUTS
- 2 TABLESPOONS FRESH CHOPPED PARSLEY (OR 1 TABLESPOON PARSLEY FLAKES)
- ½ CUP SKIM MILK
- 6 ROUND CRACKERS, CRUSHED
- SALT* AND PEPPER TO TASTE

Topping
- 4 ROUND CRACKERS, CRUSHED
- 2 TEASPOONS MARGARINE

Method

1. Preheat oven to 350° F.
2. Drain and flake tuna; add remaining ingredients and mix.
3. Pour into small loaf pan sprayed with vegetable pan spray.
4. Sprinkle crushed crackers on top of loaf; dot with margarine.
5. Bake for 1 hour. Cut into 4 slices.

Note: Tuna Loaf may be cut into 6 slices, each slice equal to:

Exchanges per slice:
    2½ Lean Meat
    ½ Bread

Estimated nutrients per serving:

CAL	179	FAT	8
CHO	5	Na	653
PRO	21	K	281

*Na content of salt not included in estimate.

Slim Chance Tuna

Yield: 5 servings
Exchanges per serving
(1 cup over ½ cup rice):
    3 Lean Meat
    2 Vegetable
  1½ Bread

Estimated nutrients per serving:

CAL	289	FAT	5
CHO	33	Na	1520*
PRO	28	K	624

Ingredients

   1 TABLESPOON MARGARINE
  ½ CUP SLICED GREEN ONIONS
   1 8-OUNCE CAN SLICED BAMBOO SHOOTS, DRAINED
   2 4-OUNCE CANS SLICED MUSHROOMS, DRAINED
   1 1-POUND CAN CHINESE VEGETABLES, DRAINED
  ⅓ CUP WATER
  ¼ TEASPOON INSTANT CHICKEN BOUILLON
   2 TEASPOONS CORNSTARCH
  ¼ TEASPOON GARLIC SALT
  ¼ TEASPOON CELERY SALT
     DASH OF PEPPER
   2 6½-OUNCE CANS WATER-PACKED TUNA, DRAINED
   1 MEDIUM TOMATO, CUT IN WEDGES
   1 CUP SHREDDED RAW SPINACH
2½ CUPS COOKED RICE
     SOY SAUCE* AS DESIRED

Method

1. Melt margarine; saute onions, bamboo shoots, and mushrooms for 2 minutes.
2. Add Chinese vegetables.

*Na content of soy sauce not included in estimate.

3. Mix together water, bouillon, cornstarch, garlic salt, celery salt, and pepper. Add to vegetables. Simmer 3 minutes.
4. Stir in tuna, tomato, and spinach. Heat through.
5. Serve over rice, with soy sauce as desired.

Salmon Soufflé

Yield: 3 cups (4 servings)
Exchanges per ¾-cup serving:
    4 Lean Meat
    ½ Bread

Estimated nutrients per serving:

CAL	269	FAT	13
CHO	8	Na	658
PRO	30	K	579

Ingredients

  1 TABLESPOON MARGARINE
  ¼ CUP SKIM MILK
  2 SLICES SOFT BREAD, CRUMBLED
  1 1-POUND CAN PINK SALMON OR MACKEREL, DRAINED AND FLAKED
  1 EGG, SEPARATED
1½ TABLESPOONS LEMON JUICE (OPTIONAL)
  1 TABLESPOON MINCED ONION
   DASH OF PEPPER
   DASH OF PAPRIKA
  2 TABLESPOONS CHOPPED FRESH PARSLEY

Method

1. Preheat oven to 325° F.
2. Mix all ingredients except egg white, paprika, and parsley.
3. Beat egg white until stiff; fold into salmon mixture.
4. Pour into 1-quart casserole sprayed with vegetable pan spray. Sprinkle with paprika and parsley.
5. Bake uncovered for 50 to 60 minutes.

Seafood Casserole

Yield: 6 servings
Exchanges per 1-cup serving:
    2 Lean Meat
    1 Vegetable
    ½ Bread
    ½ Fat

Estimated nutrients per serving:

CAL	217	FAT	9
CHO	16	Na	894
PRO	18	K	190

Ingredients

  2 6½-OUNCE CANS CRABMEAT, DRAINED AND FLAKED
  1 4½-OUNCE CAN SMALL SHRIMP, DRAINED
  1 10-OUNCE PACKAGE FROZEN PEAS, THAWED
1½ CUPS COOKED RICE
  ¼ CUP CHOPPED GREEN PEPPER
  2 TABLESPOONS CHOPPED FRESH PARSLEY
  ½ TEASPOON SALT
    PEPPER TO TASTE
  1 CUP DAIRY SOUR CREAM

Method

1. Preheat oven to 350° F.
2. Toss all ingredients together lightly.
3. Place in 2-quart casserole sprayed with vegetable pan spray.
4. Bake, covered, for 1 hour.

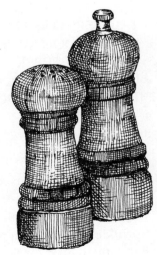

Shrimp and Mushrooms

Yield: 2⅔ cups

Exchanges per serving
(⅔ cup with ½ cup rice):

    1 Lean Meat
    2 Vegetable
    1 Bread

Estimated nutrients per serving:

CAL	208	FAT	4
CHO	29	Na	620
PRO	14	K	259

Ingredients

  1 TABLESPOON MARGARINE
1½ CUPS COOKED SHRIMP, DRAINED AND RINSED (ABOUT
    ¾ POUND FROZEN)
  ½ CUP CHOPPED CELERY
  2 TABLESPOONS MINCED ONION
  1 8-OUNCE CAN SLICED MUSHROOMS, DRAINED
  ½ CUBE BEEF BOUILLON
  ½ CUP WATER, DIVIDED
  1 TABLESPOON CORNSTARCH
  ¼ TEASPOON GINGER
    DASH PEPPER
  1 TEASPOON SOY SAUCE
  2 CUPS COOKED RICE, HOT

Method

1. In large skillet, melt margarine. Add shrimp; cook 4 to 6 minutes, stirring often.
2. Add celery, onion, and mushrooms. Cook, stirring, over high heat, 1½ to 2 minutes.
3. Dissolve bouillon cube in ¼ cup boiling water.
4. Mix cornstarch and ¼ cup cold water. Add ginger, pepper, soy sauce, and bouillon broth.
5. Pour over shrimp mixture, cooking and stirring until thick and clear. Spoon shrimp over rice.

Shrimp Creole

Yield: 4 servings

Exchanges per serving
(¾ cup over ¾ cup rice):

    2 Lean Meat
    1 Vegetable
    2 Bread

Estimated nutrients per serving:

CAL	280	FAT	8
CHO	31	Na	814
PRO	21	K	403

Ingredients

  ¼ CUP CHOPPED ONION
  ¼ CUP CHOPPED GREEN PEPPER
  1 GARLIC CLOVE, MINCED
  2 TABLESPOONS VEGETABLE OIL
  3 TABLESPOONS FLOUR
  1 TEASPOON CHILI POWDER
  1 TEASPOON SALT
    DASH OF PEPPER
  2 CUPS CANNED TOMATOES (1 16-OUNCE CAN)
2½ CUPS COOKED CLEANED SHRIMP (1 16-OUNCE BAG
    FROZEN, READY TO COOK)
  2 CUPS COOKED RICE

Method

1. Saute onion, green pepper, and garlic in oil until tender.
2. Blend in flour and seasonings.
3. Add tomato and cook until thick, stirring constantly. Simmer for 20 minutes.
4. Add shrimp. Heat through.
5. Serve over hot rice.

Main Dishes:
Egg and Cheese

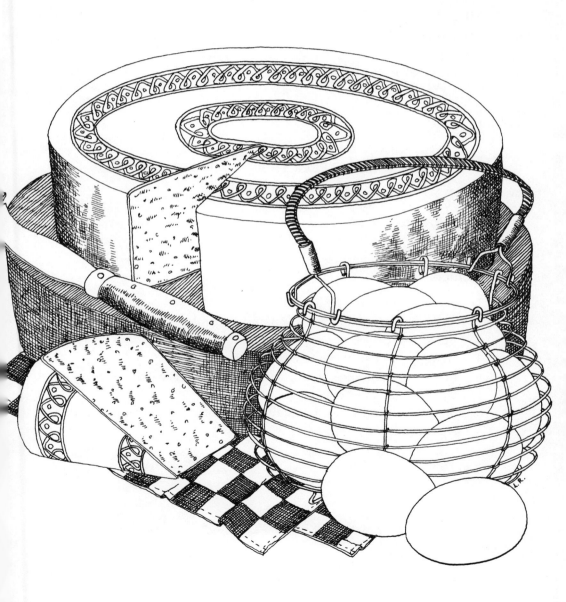

Delicious main dishes with eggs and cheeses are popular and economical for family meals. They make good choices for any meal from Sunday breakfast through family suppers.

Oven-Baked Omelet

Yield: 4 servings
Exchanges per ¼-omelet serving:

    2 Medium-Fat Meat
    1½ Fat

Estimated nutrients per serving:

CAL	225	FAT	17
CHO	3	Na	631
PRO	15	K	217

Ingredients

    4 SLICES BACON
    3 1-OUNCE SLICES PROCESSED AMERICAN CHEESE
    6 EGGS
    ¾ CUP SKIM MILK
    ¼ TEASPOON SALT
    DASH OF PEPPER

Method

1. Preheat oven to 350° F.
2. Cook bacon until crisp; drain and crumble.
3. Spray 8-inch pie pan with vegetable pan spray.
4. Arrange cheese slices to cover bottom of pan.
5. Beat together eggs, milk, salt, and pepper with a fork. Add bacon. Pour over cheese.
6. Bake for 30 minutes. Let stand 5 minutes before cutting into 4 wedges.

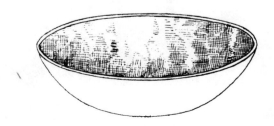

Cheese Omelet

Yield: 2 servings
Exchanges per ½-omelet
serving:

    2 Medium-Fat Meat
    1½ Fat

Estimated nutrients per serving:

CAL	218	FAT	18
CHO	—	Na	512
PRO	14	K	121

Ingredients

  3 EGGS
  1 TABLESPOON WATER
  ¼ TEASPOON SALT
    DASH OF PEPPER
  2 TEASPOONS MARGARINE
  ¼ CUP GRATED CHEDDAR CHEESE (ABOUT 1 OUNCE)

Method

1. In small bowl beat eggs, water, salt, and pepper with a fork until blended.
2. In skillet heat margarine over medium heat until it sizzles and begins to brown.
3. Remove from heat; tilt pan to coat sides.
4. Return skillet to heat. Add egg mixture and cook on medium heat without stirring. Outer edges may be lifted to allow uncooked egg to flow under when pan is tilted.
5. When omelet is set on the bottom and set but shiny on top, remove from heat. Sprinkle cheese over half of omelet. With spatula gently fold the other side over the cheese.
6. Cut into 2 servings and lift separately from pan or tilt skillet to roll omelet onto serving plate.

Variation: For Western Omelet, omit cheese and salt. Stir ¼ cup finely minced cooked ham, 2 tablespoons, chopped onion, and 2 tablespoons chopped green pepper into egg mixture before cooking. Exchanges for calories, protein, and fat are unchanged. Sodium and potassium are as follows:

Na	253
K	170

Spanish Omelet

Yield: 2 servings

Exchanges per serving
(½ omelet and ¼ cup sauce):

2 Medium-Fat Meat
1 Vegetable
1 Fat

Estimated nutrients per serving:

CAL	231	FAT	15
CHO	8	Na	1658
PRO	16	K	849

Ingredients

- 1 TEASPOON MARGARINE
- 2 TABLESPOONS CHOPPED GREEN PEPPER
- 2 TABLESPOONS CHOPPED ONION
- 2 TABLESPOONS CHOPPED CELERY
- 1 8-OUNCE CAN TOMATO SAUCE
- 1 TEASPOON WORCESTERSHIRE SAUCE
- 4 EGGS
- 2 TABLESPOONS WATER
- ½ TEASPOON SALT
- DASH OF PEPPER

Method

1. Melt margarine in skillet. Add green pepper, onion, and celery. Cook until tender. Add tomato and Worcestershire sauces. Simmer 5 to 7 minutes. Keep warm on low heat.
2. Beat eggs, water, salt, and pepper with fork.
3. Pour eggs into a second skillet sprayed with vegetable pan spray.
4. Cook on medium heat without stirring. Outer edges may be lifted to allow uncooked egg to flow under when pan is tilted.
5. When eggs are brown on bottom, spoon ½ cup of sauce over half of the omelet. With spatula fold other side of omelet over the sauce.
6. Cut into two servings and lift separately from pan or tilt skillet to roll omelet onto serving plate.
7. Spoon half of the remaining sauce over each serving.

Scrambled Egg and Ham Supper

Yield: 4 servings
Exchanges per ¾-cup serving:
    2 High-Fat Meat

Estimated nutrients per serving:

CAL	195	FAT	15
CHO	1	Na	735
PRO	14	K	201

Ingredients

  6 EGGS
  5 RIPE OLIVES, SLICED
  1 TABLESPOON MINCED ONION
 ¼ CUP CHOPPED GREEN PEPPER
 ½ TEASPOON SALT
    DASH OF PEPPER
 ½ CUP DICED COOKED HAM (ABOUT 2 OUNCES)
  1 TABLESPOON MARGARINE.

Method

1. Beat eggs in bowl. Add all other ingredients except margarine.
2. Melt margarine in skillet.
3. Add egg mixture. Cook, stirring gently, until eggs are cooked throughout but still moist.

Spinach Quiche

Yield: 6 servings
Exchanges per 1/6-wedge
serving:
   ½ Milk
    1 High-Fat Meat
    1 Vegetable
 1½ Bread
    3 Fat

Estimated nutrients per serving:

CAL	421	FAT	25
CHO	33	Na	734
PRO	16	K	470

Ingredients

1½ CUPS SIFTED FLOUR
½ TEASPOON SALT
½ CUP VEGETABLE SHORTENING
3 TABLESPOONS ICE WATER
1 10-OUNCE PACKAGE FROZEN CHOPPED SPINACH
4 GREEN ONIONS WITH TOPS, SLICED
4 EGGS
1 13-OUNCE CAN EVAPORATED SKIM MILK
¼ TEASPOON DRY MUSTARD
½ TEASPOON SALT
⅛ TEASPOON PEPPER
½ CUP GRATED PARMESAN CHEESE

Method

1. Combine flour, salt, and shortening in medium bowl. Mix lightly with fingers or pastry blender until texture of soft bread crumbs. Sprinkle ice water over dough. Toss gently until dough will form a ball. If it's too dry, add 1 tablespoon ice water. Wrap dough in wax paper and chill 1 hour.
2. Preheat oven to 400° F. Remove dough from refrigerator. Let stand 5 minutes before rolling. Roll dough into a circle on lightly floured board or between sheets of wax paper. Fit dough into 9-inch pie pan; flute rim. Prick crust with fork tines about 8 times. Bake 10 minutes or until shell is lightly browned. Remove from oven and let cool.
3. Cook spinach until tender. Drain very thoroughly.
4. Beat eggs. Add spinach and remaining ingredients except cheese.
5. Sprinkle half of Parmesan cheese on pie shell. Pour filling in crust. Sprinkle top of pie with remaining cheese.
6. Bake in 400° F oven 30 to 35 minutes or until knife inserted in the center comes out clean. Remove from oven. Let stand 10 minutes before cutting into 6 servings.

Eggs Goldenrod

Yield: 6 servings
Exchanges per serving (scant
½ cup on 1 slice toast):

    1 Medium-Fat Meat
  1½ Bread
    1 Fat

Estimated nutrients per serving:

CAL	214	FAT	10
CHO	21	Na	469
PRO	10	K	211

Ingredients

  4 HARD-COOKED EGGS
  3 TABLESPOONS MARGARINE
  3 TABLESPOONS FLOUR
  2 CUPS SKIM MILK
  ¼ TEASPOON DRY MUSTARD
  ½ TEASPOON SALT
    PEPPER TO TASTE
  6 SLICES BREAD, TOASTED

Method

1. Chop eggs, reserving 2 yolks for garnish.
2. In saucepan melt margarine over low heat. Blend in flour and seasonings.
3. Add milk, stirring constantly. Remove from heat when sauce thickens and bubbles.
4. Add chopped eggs. Heat.
5. Serve on toast. Force 2 egg yolks through a sieve to garnish.

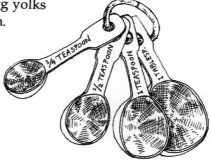

Macaroni and Cheese Custard

Yield: 6 servings
Exchanges per ¾-cup serving:
    2 Medium-Fat Meat
    1½ Bread
    ½ Fat

Estimated nutrients per serving:

CAL	257	FAT	13
CHO	18	Na	1084
PRO	17	K	221

Ingredients

1½ QUARTS WATER
1½ TEASPOONS SALT
  1 CUP UNCOOKED ELBOW MACARONI
  1 TEASPOON MARGARINE
  2 CUPS SKIM MILK
  1 TEASPOON SALT
 ⅛ TEASPOON PEPPER
1½ CUPS GRATED SHARP CHEDDAR CHEESE (ABOUT
    6 OUNCES)
  3 EGGS, BEATEN
  1 TABLESPOON CHOPPED FRESH PARSLEY

Method

1. Bring salted water to a boil. Add macaroni and cook, stirring occasionally, 10 minutes or until tender.
2. Preheat oven to 325° F.
3. Drain macaroni and return to saucepan. Add margarine, stir to coat macaroni.
4. Add remaining ingredients; mix well.
5. Pour into baking dish. Bake in oven 1 hour. Let stand 10 minutes before serving.

Deviled Eggs

Yield: 4 servings
Exchanges per 2-halves
serving:

    1 Medium-Fat Meat
  ½ Fat

Estimated nutrients per serving:

CAL	95	FAT	7
CHO	1	Na	172*
PRO	7	K	78

Ingredients

   4 HARD-COOKED EGGS
   4 TEASPOONS DAIRY SOUR CREAM
   2 TEASPOONS PREPARED MUSTARD
   2 TEASPOONS VINEGAR
     SALT* AND PEPPER TO TASTE
     DASH OF PAPRIKA

Method

1. Slice eggs in half lengthwise.
2. Remove egg yolks; mash with a fork.
3. Add sour cream, mustard, vinegar, salt, and pepper. Mix well until smooth.
4. Fill egg whites with yolk mixture. Garnish with a dash of paprika.

*Na content of salt not included in estimate.

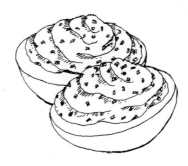

Creamy Macaroni and Cheese

Yield: 4 servings
Exchanges per 1-cup serving:
    2 Medium-Fat Meat
   1½ Bread
    1 Fat

Estimated nutrients per serving:

CAL	317	FAT	17
CHO	24	Na	634
PRO	17	K	300

Ingredients

   2 CUPS COOKED ELBOW MACARONI (1 CUP UNCOOKED)
   2 TABLESPOONS GRATED ONION
1½ CUPS GRATED CHEDDAR CHEESE (ABOUT 6 OUNCES)
   1 TABLESPOON MARGARINE
   1 TABLESPOON FLOUR
   2 CUPS SKIM MILK
  ½ TEASPOON SALT
  ¼ TEASPOON PEPPER

Method

1. Preheat oven to 375° F.
2. Place half of the cooked macaroni in a 1½-quart casserole sprayed with vegetable pan spray. Sprinkle with half of onion and cheese. Repeat layers.
3. Melt margarine in small saucepan. Remove from heat, stir in flour. Add milk slowly, stirring until smooth. Add salt and pepper. Return pan to heat; cook, stirring constantly, until sauce thickens. (This will be a thin sauce.)
4. Pour over macaroni. Cover. Bake for 30 minutes. Uncover. Bake 15 minutes longer.

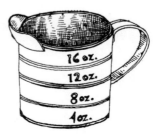

Cheese Timbales

Yield: 6 timbales

Exchanges per 1-timbale serving:

    1½ Medium-Fat Meat
    ½ Bread
    1 Fat

Estimated nutrients per serving:

CAL	192	FAT	12
CHO	9	Na	629
PRO	12	K	221

Ingredients

- 2 CUPS SKIM MILK
- 1 TABLESPOON MARGARINE
- 2 SLICES BREAD, CRUMBLED
- 1 TEASPOON SALT
- ½ TEASPOON DRY MUSTARD
- 1 TEASPOON MINCED CHIVES
- ¼ TEASPOON PEPPER
- 1 CUP GRATED CHEDDAR CHEESE (ABOUT 4 OUNCES), DIVIDED
- 3 EGGS, LIGHTLY BEATEN

Method

1. Scald milk with margarine.
2. Add bread crumbs. Let stand 15 minutes.
3. Preheat oven to 350° F.
4. Add all remaining ingredients except 2 tablespoons cheese.
5. Spray 6-ounce custard cups with vegetable pan spray. Put 1 teaspoon reserved cheese in each cup. Pour ½ cup egg mixture over cheese.
6. Place cups in pan of hot water. Bake for about 1½ hours, or until knife inserted in center comes out clean.
7. Let stand 5 minutes. Unmold to serve.

Serving suggestion: Serve with Mushroom Sauce (see index) if desired.

Shrimp Egg Foo Yung

Yield: 4 servings

Exchanges per serving (¼ recipe with 2 tablespoons sauce):

    2 Medium-Fat Meat
    1 Vegetable
  2½ Fat

Estimated nutrients per serving:

CAL	295	FAT	23
CHO	8	Na	748
PRO	14	K	283

Ingredients

  6 MEDIUM EGGS
 ½ TEASPOON SALT
 ⅓ CUP SMALL (OR DICED) COOKED SHRIMP
  3 TABLESPOONS FINELY CHOPPED CELERY
  1 CUP BEAN SPROUTS
  3 TABLESPOONS FINELY SLIVERED WATER CHESTNUTS
 ⅓ CUP THINLY SLICED MUSHROOMS
 ¼ CUP VEGETABLE OIL

Sauce

 ½ CUP WATER
  1 TABLESPOON CORNSTARCH
  1 TEASPOON SOY SAUCE
  1 BEEF BOUILLON CUBE

Method

1. Beat eggs and salt until light and fluffy.
2. Add shrimp, celery, bean sprouts, water chestnuts, and mushrooms.

3. Heat 1 tablespoon oil in small skillet. Pour into skillet ½ cup of mixture (¼ of recipe). Cook over medium heat until brown, then turn and brown on the other side.

4. Repeat procedure for other 3 servings. Top with hot egg foo yung sauce.

Sauce

1. Blend water with cornstarch.
2. Add soy sauce and bouillon cube.
3. Cook over medium heat until sauce thickens. Serve hot.

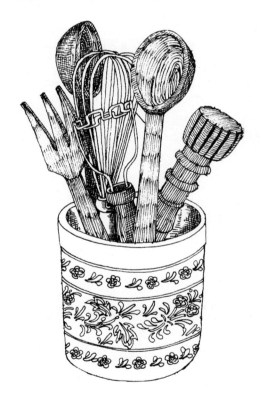

Rice and Pasta Dishes

The Bread Exchange on the meal plan need not always be a slice of
bread. Provide variations with pasta or rice cooked in new ways.

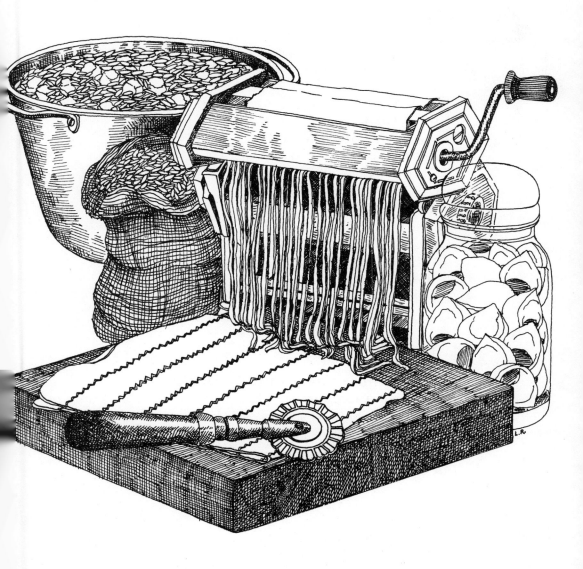

Lasagne

Yield: 12 servings, 3 × 4 inches each square

Exchanges per single serving:

   3 Lean Meat
1½ Bread
   1 Fat

Estimated nutrients per serving:

CAL	322	FAT	14
CHO	23	Na	852
PRO	26	K	650

Ingredients

   1 POUND GROUND BEEF
  ¾ CUP CHOPPED ONION
   1 CLOVE GARLIC, PEELED AND CRUSHED
   1 16-OUNCE CAN TOMATOES
1½ CUPS TOMATO PASTE (2 6-OUNCE CANS)
   2 TEASPOONS BASIL
   1 TEASPOON OREGANO
   2 TEASPOONS SALT
   8 OUNCES LASAGNE NOODLES
   3 CUPS LOW-FAT COTTAGE CHEESE
   1 TABLESPOON PARSLEY FLAKES
   2 EGGS, BEATEN
  ¾ POUND SHREDDED MOZZARELLA CHEESE
  ½ CUP GRATED PARMESAN CHEESE

Method

1. Brown beef with onion and garlic. Drain.
2. Add tomatoes, tomato paste, basil, oregano, and salt. Simmer uncovered 30 minutes, stirring occasionally.
3. Preheat oven to 350° F.
4. Cook lasagne noodles according to package instructions.
5. Mix cottage cheese, parsley flakes, and eggs.

6. In 9- × 13-inch baking pan, layer half the noodles, cottage cheese mixture, and meat sauce. Repeat layers with remaining ingredients. Sprinkle with Parmesan cheese.
7. Bake for 45 minutes. Let stand 10 minutes before cutting into 12 squares (about 3 × 4 inches).

Spanish Tomato Rice

Yield: 3 cups
Exchanges per ¾-cup serving:
  1 Vegetable
  2 Bread
  1 Fat

Estimated nutrients per serving:

CAL	204	FAT	4
CHO	36	Na	1209
PRO	6	K	506

Ingredients

  4 SLICES BACON
  1 CUP CHOPPED ONION
  ¼ CUP CHOPPED GREEN PEPPER
  1 16-OUNCE CAN TOMATOES
1½ CUPS WATER
  ¾ CUP UNCOOKED RICE
  ½ CUP CHILI SAUCE
  1 TEASPOON SALT
    DASH OF PEPPER
  1 TEASPOON BROWN SUGAR
  ½ TEASPOON WORCESTERSHIRE SAUCE
  2 TABLESPOONS CHOPPED FRESH PARSLEY

Method

1. Cook bacon until crisp. Drain on paper towels. Drain fat from skillet, reserving 1 tablespoon of fat.
2. Brown onion and green pepper in the reserved fat until tender.
3. Add remaining ingredients except bacon and parsley. Simmer 45 minutes.
4. Crumble bacon on top and sprinkle with chopped parsley before serving.

Pork Sausage Casserole

Yield: 8 servings
Exchanges per 1-cup serving:
    1 High-Fat Meat
    ½ Vegetable
    1½ Bread
    1½ Fat

Estimated nutrients per serving:

CAL	283	FAT	15
CHO	25	Na	606
PRO	12	K	365

Ingredients

    1 POUND BULK PORK SAUSAGE
    ½ CUP CHOPPED GREEN PEPPER
    8 OUNCES FINE NOODLES, UNCOOKED
    1 28-OUNCE CAN TOMATOES, MASHED (UNDRAINED)
    6 BAY LEAVES
    DASH PAPRIKA
    ½ TEASPOON WORCESTERSHIRE SAUCE
    ½ CUP GRATED PARMESAN CHEESE

Method

1. Preheat oven to 350° F.
2. Crumble sausage and cook slowly with green pepper until brown. Remove from heat; drain well.
3. Cook noodles in boiling salted water. Drain; turn into 2-quart casserole. Add sausage and pepper.
4. Simmer remaining ingredients except the cheese in saucepan for 5 minutes, stirring occasionally. Remove bay leaves. Add remaining mixture to sausage. Mix well. Shake Parmesan cheese over top.
5. Bake uncovered 35 to 40 minutes.

Tomato Soup Casserole

Yield: 6 cups

Exchanges per 1-cup serving:

   2 Medium-Fat Meat

   2 Bread

Estimated nutrients per serving:

CAL	292	FAT	12
CHO	28	Na	984
PRO	18	K	483

Ingredients

  ⅔ CUP LONG GRAIN RICE, UNCOOKED
  1 POUND GROUND BEEF
  ½ CUP CHOPPED ONION
  ¾ TEASPOON SALT
  ¼ TEASPOON PAPRIKA
  1 CUP CHOPPED CELERY
  ¼ CUP CHOPPED GREEN PEPPER
  1 10¾-OUNCE CAN TOMATO SOUP, CONDENSED
  ½ CUP WATER

Method

1. Cook rice according to package directions.
2. Preheat oven to 350° F.
3. Brown ground beef and onion in skillet. Drain. Season with salt and paprika.
4. Combine meat mixture with rice and remaining ingredients in 2-quart casserole; cover.
5. Bake for 30 minutes.

Wild Rice and Mushrooms

Yield: 4 cups
Exchanges per ½-cup serving:
   1 Bread
   ½ Fat

Estimated nutrients per serving:

CAL	94	FAT	2
CHO	17	Na	416
PRO	2	K	80

Ingredients

  1 TABLESPOON MARGARINE
  1 CUP FINELY CHOPPED ONION
  1 4-OUNCE CAN MUSHROOM STEMS AND PIECES, DRAINED
  2 CHICKEN BOUILLON CUBES
2½ CUPS WATER
  1 6-OUNCE BOX LONG GRAIN AND WILD RICE
  2 TABLESPOONS MINCED FRESH PARSLEY
   (OR 1 TABLESPOON PARSLEY FLAKES)

Method

1. Melt margarine in saucepan. Saute onion until clear.
2. Add remaining ingredients. Bring to a boil.
3. Cover. Reduce heat and cook 25 to 30 minutes, until water is absorbed.

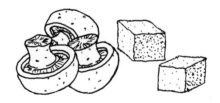

Cheese 'n' Rice Stuffed Pepper

Yield: 2 servings
Exchanges per 1-pepper serving:
    1 Medium-Fat Meat
   1½ Bread
    1 Fat

Estimated nutrients per serving:

CAL	234	FAT	10
CHO	25	Na	743
PRO	11	K	445

Ingredients

  2 GREEN PEPPERS, MEDIUM
  ½ CUP GRATED CHEDDAR CHEESE (ABOUT 2 OUNCES)
  1 CUP COOKED RICE
  ¼ TEASPOON SALT
    DASH PEPPER

Method

1. Preheat oven to 300° F.
2. Slice off tops of green peppers. Wash peppers and remove seeds. Stand pepper cups upright in saucepan containing ½ cup boiling water. Cover and steam 5 minutes. Drain.
3. Mix together cheese, rice, salt, and pepper.
4. Fill each pepper with half of cheese mixture.
5. Stand peppers in loaf pan. Bake for 10 or 15 minutes until cheese melts.

Variation: Cook rice in tomato juice or broth instead of water. Add 2 tablespoons chopped onion or fresh parsley in Step 3.

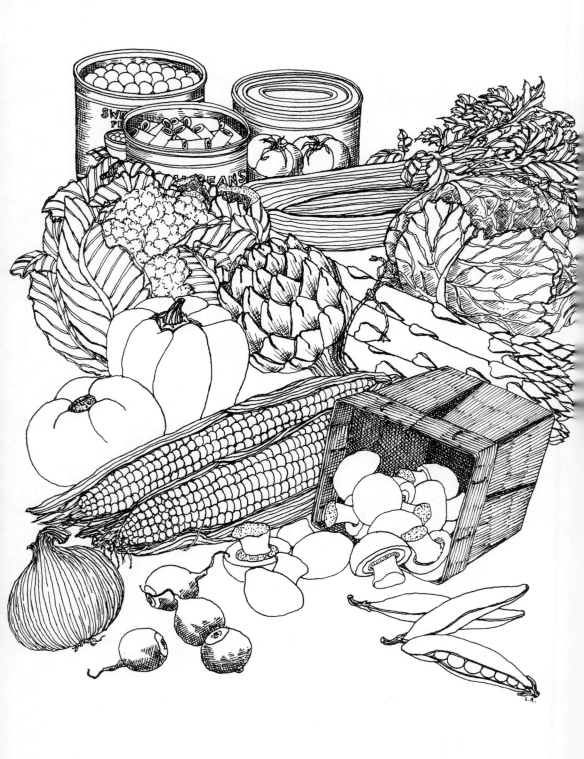

Vegetables

A well-chosen, well-cooked vegetable adds color, texture, and flavor to the meal. With the choice of fresh, canned, and frozen vegetables available year-round you can offer the family enough variety to please everyone.

When recipes were being home-tested for this section of the cookbook, it was heartening to note that many people commented that they like their vegetables plain. Vegetables cooked until just tender and nicely seasoned are always appealing. The recipes in this section offer variations to entice you to introduce the family to some vegetables you may not have served before.

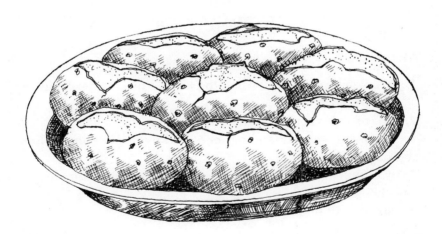

Cheesy Asparagus Crepes

Yield: 12 crepes

Exchanges per 2-crepe serving:

   ½ Medium-Fat Meat

   1 Vegetable

   1 Bread

   1 Fat

Estimated nutrients per serving:

CAL	180	FAT	8
CHO	19	Na	321*
PRO	8	K	300

Ingredients

  2 8-OUNCE PACKAGES FROZEN ASPARAGUS SPEARS

12 PREPARED BASIC CREPES (SEE INDEX)

    SALT* TO TASTE

    PEPPER TO TASTE

 ½ 10½-OUNCE CAN CREAM OF MUSHROOM SOUP, UNDILUTED

  2 TABLESPOONS SKIM MILK

 ¼ CUP GRATED CHEDDAR CHEESE (1 OUNCE)

Method

1. Cook asparagus according to package directions; drain thoroughly.
2. Place stalks across center of each crepe.
3. Sprinkle with salt and pepper. Fold over. Place in shallow baking pan.
4. Combine soup and milk. Spoon over crepes. Sprinkle with cheese.
5. Broil until bubbly.

*Na content of salt not included in estimate.

Spinach Crepes

Yield: 8 crepes
Exchanges per 2-crepe serving:
    2 Medium-Fat Meat
    ½ Vegetable
    1 Bread
    ½ Fat

Estimated nutrients per serving:

CAL	257	FAT	13
CHO	19	Na	413
PRO	16	K	456

Ingredients

  1 10-OUNCE PACKAGE FROZEN CHOPPED SPINACH
 ¼ TEASPOON SALT
    DASH PEPPER
 ½ CUP RICOTTA CHEESE
  3 TABLESPOONS EVAPORATED SKIM MILK
  2 EGGS, SLIGHTLY BEATEN
    DASH NUTMEG
  8 PREPARED BASIC CREPES (SEE INDEX)
  2 TEASPOONS MARGARINE, MELTED
  3 TABLESPOONS GRATED PARMESAN CHEESE

Method

1. Preheat oven to 350° F.
2. Cook spinach according to package directions. Drain thoroughly.
3. Add salt, pepper, ricotta cheese, milk, eggs, and nutmeg.
4. Put ¼ cup filling in center of each crepe; overlap sides.
5. Place seam side down in 13- × 9-inch baking dish. Brush with margarine. Sprinkle with Parmesan cheese.
6. Heat for 20 minutes.

Snappy Green Beans

Yield: 2 cups

Estimated nutrients per serving:

Exchanges per ½-cup serving:

	CAL	64	FAT	4
1 Vegetable	CHO	5	Na	157
1 Fat	PRO	2	K	117

Ingredients

- 1½ CUPS CUT GREEN BEANS (OR 1 9-OUNCE PACKAGE FROZEN)
- ¼ CUP CHOPPED ONION
- 1 TEASPOON MARGARINE
- 1½ TEASPOONS FLOUR
- ¼ TEASPOON SALT
- DASH OF PEPPER
- ¼ CUP WATER
- 1½ TEASPOONS VINEGAR
- 1 TABLESPOON CHOPPED PIMIENTO
- ⅛ TEASPOON DILL WEED
- ¼ CUP DAIRY SOUR CREAM

Method

1. Cook green beans in ½ cup water until barely tender. Drain.
2. In saucepan, cook onion in margarine until tender. Stir in flour, salt, and pepper.
3. Add water, vinegar, pimiento, and dill weed. Cook, stirring until bubbly.
4. Stir in sour cream. Add green beans.
5. Heat mixture through but do not boil.

Barbecue Limas

Yield: 4 cups
Exchanges per ½-cup serving:

    1 Vegetable
    1 Bread
    ½ Fruit

Estimated nutrients per serving:

CAL	116	FAT	1
CHO	23	Na	215
PRO	6	K	486

Ingredients

1¼ CUPS DRY LIMA BEANS (½ POUND)
  1 HAM BONE
 ½ MEDIUM ONION, SLICED
 ½ TEASPOON SALT
 ¼ TEASPOON DRY MUSTARD
 ½ TEASPOON VINEGAR
  2 TABLESPOONS MOLASSES
  3 TABLESPOONS CHILI SAUCE

Method

1. Place beans in soup pot with ham bone. Add 3 cups water. Boil 2 minutes; remove from heat; cover; let stand 1 hour.
2. Preheat oven to 300° F.
3. Drain beans, reserving 1 cup liquid. Combine beans and reserved liquid with remaining ingredients.
4. Bake in 1½-quart casserole for 2¼ hours, uncovering last 30 minutes. More liquid may be added if necessary.

Red Beans and Rice

Yield: 6 servings
Exchanges per serving (scant
½ cup beans over ¼ cup rice):

    ½ Lean Meat
    2 Bread

Estimated nutrients per serving:

CAL	173	FAT	1
CHO	32	Na	324
PRO	9	K	354

Ingredients

1¼ CUPS DRY RED KIDNEY BEANS (8 OUNCES)
  1 HAM BONE
  1 ONION, CHOPPED
  1 BAY LEAF
 ½ TEASPOON SALT
 ¼ TEASPOON TABASCO SAUCE
1½ CUPS HOT COOKED RICE

Method

1. Place beans in soup pot with 5 cups water. Boil 2 minutes; cover; let stand 1 hour.
2. Add remaining ingredients except rice. Simmer 1 hour or until beans are tender. Remove ham bone and bay leaf.
3. Remove ½ cup beans and mash. Return to pot; heat, stirring, until liquid is thickened.
4. Serve beans over hot cooked rice.

Boston Baked Beans

Yield: 3 cups

Exchanges per ½-cup serving:
 1 Medium-Fat Meat
 1 Bread
 1 Fruit

Estimated nutrients per serving:

CAL	181	FAT	5
CHO	25	Na	184
PRO	9	K	687

Ingredients

 1 CUP DRY NAVY BEANS (APPROXIMATELY ½ POUND)
 ¼ TEASPOON SALT
 3 TABLESPOONS DARK MOLASSES
 ½ TEASPOON DRY MUSTARD
 6 SLICES BACON, CUT IN HALF
 ½ MEDIUM ONION, CHOPPED

Method

1. Rinse beans. Add to 1 quart cold water. Bring to boil; simmer 2 minutes. Remove from heat. Cover; let stand 1 hour.
2. Add salt. Cover; simmer 1 hour. Drain, reserving 1 cup of liquid. (Add water if necessary to make 1 cup.) Add molasses and mustard to liquid.
3. Preheat oven to 300° F.
4. In 1-quart casserole combine beans, bacon, and onion. Pour liquid over beans.
5. Cover, bake 3 to 4 hours.

Harvard Beets

Yield: 2½ cups
Exchanges per ½-cup serving:
   1 Vegetable
   ½ Fruit

Estimated nutrients per serving:

CAL	44	FAT	—
CHO	10	Na	378
PRO	1	K	116

Ingredients

   1 1-POUND CAN BEETS, SLICED (SAVE LIQUID)
   1 TABLESPOON CORNSTARCH
  ½ TEASPOON SALT
    DASH OF PEPPER
  ¼ CUP VINEGAR
   1 TABLESPOON SUGAR

Method

1. Drain beets, reserving liquid. Add enough water to beet juice to make ⅔ cup liquid.
2. Combine cornstarch, salt, and pepper in saucepan. Add liquid and vinegar. Stir until smooth.
3. Cook, stirring constantly, until mixture thickens and boils. Boil 1 minute, stirring.
4. Add sliced beets and sugar; heat through.

Broccoli au Gratin

Yield: 2 cups

Estimated nutrients per serving:

Exchanges per ½-cup serving:

2 Vegetable	
1 Fat	

CAL	102	FAT	6
CHO	8	Na	368
PRO	4	K	159

Ingredients

- 1 10-OUNCE PACKAGE FROZEN BROCCOLI, CUTS OR CHOPPED
- ½ 10½-OUNCE CAN CREAM OF MUSHROOM SOUP
- ¼ CUP GRATED CHEDDAR CHEESE (ABOUT 1 OUNCE)
- 1 TEASPOON MARGARINE
- 2 TABLESPOONS DRY BREAD CRUMBS

Method

1. Preheat oven to 350° F.
2. Cook broccoli until crisp-tender. Drain.
3. Stir in soup and cheese. Turn into 1-quart baking dish.
4. Melt margarine in small skillet over medium heat. Add bread crumbs; stir until lightly browned. Sprinkle over casserole.
5. Bake 25 to 30 minutes or until heated through.

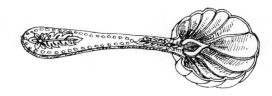

Broccoli-Potato Bake

Yield: 4 cups

Exchanges per 1-cup serving:

    1 Vegetable

    1 Bread

    1 Fat

Estimated nutrients per serving:

CAL	153	FAT	5
CHO	20	Na	639
PRO	7	K	539

Ingredients

    4 SMALL POTATOES, PEELED AND DICED

    2 TEASPOONS MARGARINE

    1 TEASPOON SALT

    ¼ CUP SKIM MILK

    1 10-OUNCE PACKAGE FROZEN CHOPPED BROCCOLI

    ¼ CUP GRATED CHEDDAR CHEESE (ABOUT 1 OUNCE)

Method

1. Cook, drain, and mash potatoes with margarine, salt, and milk.
2. Preheat oven to 350° F.
3. Cook broccoli according to package directions. Drain well. Fold into mashed potatoes.
4. Put in casserole sprayed with vegetable pan spray. Sprinkle with cheese.
5. Bake for 15 minutes or until cheese melts.

Sweet 'n' Sour Brussels Sprouts

Yield: 1½ cups

Exchanges per ½-cup serving:
    1½ Vegetable
    ½ Fat

Estimated nutrients per serving:

CAL	75	FAT	3
CHO	8	Na	424
PRO	4	K	245

Ingredients

1½ CUPS BRUSSELS SPROUTS (1 9-OUNCE PACKAGE FROZEN)
  2 SLICES BACON
  2 TABLESPOONS VINEGAR
1½ TEASPOONS SUGAR
  ½ TEASPOON SALT
  ¼ TEASPOON GARLIC POWDER

Method

1. Cook brussels sprouts according to package directions. Drain thoroughly.
2. Fry bacon until crisp. Drain; crumble.
3. Combine vinegar, sugar, and seasonings. Stir into sprouts.
4. Sprinkle bacon over sprouts. Heat through.

Crisp Red Cabbage

Yield: 3 cups

Exchanges per ½-cup serving:
  1 Vegetable
  1 Fruit

Estimated nutrients per serving:

CAL	67	FAT	1
CHO	15	Na	105
PRO	1	K	202

Ingredients

  4 CUPS SHREDDED RED CABBAGE (ABOUT ¾ POUND)
  2 MEDIUM APPLES, CORED AND CUT INTO WEDGES
  ¼ CUP RED WINE VINEGAR
  2 TABLESPOONS BROWN SUGAR
  ¼ TEASPOON SALT
  ¼ TEASPOON GROUND NUTMEG

Method

1. Place cabbage, apples, vinegar, and brown sugar in saucepan over medium heat. Mix well.
2. Cover, simmer about 10 minutes until cabbage is tender-crisp.
3. Add salt and nutmeg. Mix well. Serve warm.

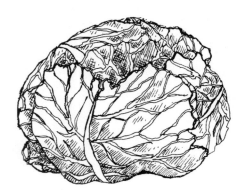

Orange Glazed Carrots

Yield: 3 cups
Exchanges per ½-cup serving:
    1 Vegetable
    1 Fat
    ½ Fruit

Estimated nutrients per serving:

CAL	84	FAT	4
CHO	10	Na	250
PRO	2	K	243

Ingredients

  ½ CUP WATER
  ½ TEASPOON SALT
2½ CUPS SLICED CARROTS
  ½ CUP UNSWEETENED ORANGE JUICE
  1 TABLESPOON CORNSTARCH
  2 TABLESPOONS MARGARINE
  1 MEDIUM ORANGE, DICED OR SECTIONED

Method

1. Bring salted water to boil. Add carrots; cover and cook until barely tender.
2. Drain the liquid into measuring cup. Add orange juice. Add enough water to make 1 cup of liquid.
3. Remove carrots from pan.
4. In saucepan mix liquids with cornstarch. Cook on medium heat, stirring constantly, until thickened and clear.
5. Add margarine, carrots, and oranges; heat through.

Cauliflower Supreme

Yield: 2½ cups
Exchanges per ½-cup serving:
   1 Vegetable
   ½ Fat
   ½ Fruit

Estimated nutrients per serving:

CAL	78	FAT	2
CHO	12	Na	222
PRO	3	K	169

Ingredients

   1 SMALL HEAD CAULIFLOWER
   ¾ CUP BOILING WATER
   ½ TEASPOON SALT
   1 CUP SEEDLESS GRAPES, HALVED
   2 TABLESPOONS TOASTED ALMONDS

Method

1. Break off flowerets of cauliflower; slice lengthwise into ¼-inch thick slices.
2. Simmer cauliflower in boiling water in covered pan 5 minutes or until tender; remove from heat; drain.
3. Fold in grapes and almonds.
4. Return to burner until heated through.

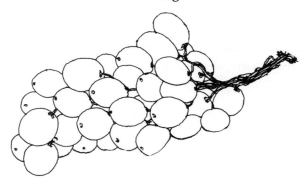

Scalloped Corn

Yield: 4 cups
Exchanges per ½-cup serving:
    ½ Milk
    1 Bread
    ½ Fat

Estimated nutrients per serving:

CAL	135	FAT	3
CHO	22	Na	328
PRO	5	K	134

Ingredients

  1 17-OUNCE CAN CREAM STYLE CORN
  1 CUP SKIM MILK
  1 EGG, BEATEN
  1 CUP CRACKER CRUMBS, DIVIDED
  2 TABLESPOONS CHOPPED PIMIENTO
  ¼ CUP CHOPPED ONION
  ½ TEASPOON SALT
    DASH OF PEPPER
  1 TEASPOON MARGARINE

Method

1. Preheat oven to 350° F.
2. Combine corn and milk. Stir in egg.
3. Add ¾ cup of crumbs, pimiento, onion, salt, and pepper. Mix well.
4. Pour into 1-quart baking dish sprayed with vegetable pan spray.
5. Melt margarine in small skillet. Add remaining ¼ cup cracker crumbs; stir until lightly browned. Spread over corn mixture.
6. Bake for 45 minutes.

Succotash

Yield: 3 cups
Exchanges per ½-cup serving:
    1 Bread
    ½ Fat

Estimated nutrients per serving:

CAL	82	FAT	2
CHO	13	Na	279*
PRO	3	K	124

Ingredients

  1 12-OUNCE CAN WHOLE KERNEL CORN, DRAINED
  1 1-POUND CAN LIMA BEANS, DRAINED
  ⅓ CUP DAIRY SOUR CREAM
    SALT* AND PEPPER TO TASTE

Method

1. Combine all ingredients.
2. Heat over medium heat until it begins to bubble.

*Na content of salt not included in estimate.

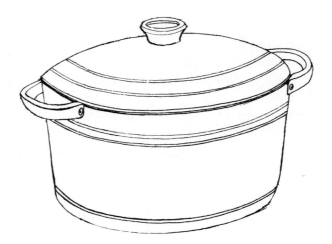

Eggplant Parmesan

Yield: 3 cups

Exchanges per ½-cup serving:

    1 Medium-Fat Meat

    1 Vegetable

Estimated nutrients per serving:

CAL	97	FAT	5
CHO	8	Na	242*
PRO	5	K	329

Ingredients

    1 MEDIUM EGGPLANT, PEELED AND SLICED

    1 CUP STEWED TOMATOES

  ¼ CUP BREAD CRUMBS

      SALT* TO TASTE

      PEPPER TO TASTE

      OREGANO TO TASTE

  ½ CUP TOMATO SAUCE

  ¾ CUP GRATED CHEDDAR CHEESE (3 OUNCES)

    3 TABLESPOONS PARMESAN CHEESE

Method

1. Simmer eggplant in pan of boiling, salted water for 10 minutes. Drain.
2. Preheat oven to 350° F.
3. Layer ingredients in 1½-quart casserole as follows: one-half of tomatoes, eggplant, bread crumbs, seasonings, tomato sauce, and cheeses. Repeat layers.
4. Bake, uncovered, for 20 minutes.

*Na content of salt not included in estimate.

Ratatouille

Yield: 4 cups
Exchanges per ½-cup serving:

  2 Vegetable
  1 Fat

Estimated nutrients per serving:

CAL	102	FAT	6
CHO	9	Na	42
PRO	3	K	381

Ingredients

  2 MEDIUM TOMATOES, CUT IN WEDGES
  ⅛ TEASPOON THYME
  1 TEASPOON SALT
  1 MEDIUM ONION, SLICED
  1 MEDIUM GREEN PEPPER, CUT IN STRIPS
  2 CUPS EGGPLANT, PEELED, SLICED AND CUT IN STRIPS
  2 CUPS ZUCCHINI, SLICED AND CUT IN STRIPS
  2 GARLIC CLOVES, CRUSHED
  3 TABLESPOONS VEGETABLE OIL
  ½ BAY LEAF
    PEPPER TO TASTE
  3 TABLESPOONS GRATED PARMESAN CHEESE

Method

1. Preheat oven to 350° F.
2. Sprinkle tomatoes with thyme and salt. Let stand.
3. Saute remaining vegetables and garlic in oil until barely tender. Add bay leaf.
4. Turn into 1½-quart casserole. Arrange tomato wedges on top. Sprinkle with pepper and cheese.
5. Bake, covered, for 30 minutes. Remove bay leaf before serving.

Pan-Fried Onions

Yield: 2 cups

Exchanges per ½-cup serving:
    1 Vegetable
    1 Fat

Estimated nutrients per serving:

CAL	64	FAT	4
CHO	6	Na	279
PRO	1	K	118

Ingredients

    3 MEDIUM ONIONS
    1 TABLESPOON VEGETABLE OIL
    ½ TEASPOON SALT

Method

1. Slice onions thinly and separate into rings. (Makes about 3 cups onion rings.)
2. Heat oil in skillet.
3. Add onions and salt. Toss in pan to coat with oil. Cook about 10 minutes over medium heat, stirring often, until crisp-tender and lightly browned.

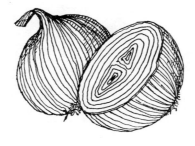

Green Peas Oriental

Yield: 3 cups

Exchanges per ¾-cup serving:
  1 Vegetable
  1 Bread
  1 Fat

Estimated nutrients per serving:

CAL	138	FAT	6
CHO	16	Na	680
PRO	5	K	182

Ingredients

    1 10-OUNCE PACKAGE FROZEN PEAS, THAWED
    3 WATER CHESTNUTS, SLICED
    1 4-OUNCE CAN MUSHROOM STEMS AND PIECES,
       DRAINED
    1 10½-OUNCE CAN CREAM OF MUSHROOM SOUP

Method

1. Preheat oven to 350° F.
2. Combine all ingredients.
3. Pour into 1-quart baking dish. Cover. Bake for 30 minutes.

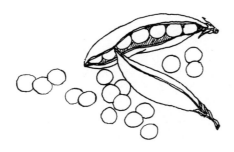

Rutabaga in Potato Nest

Yield: 6 cups
Exchanges per serving (½ cup
potato and ½ cup rutabaga)

    1 Vegetable
    1 Bread
    1 Fat

Estimated nutrients per serving:

CAL	136	FAT	4
CHO	22	Na	60*
PRO	3	K	465

Ingredients

    5 SMALL POTATOES
    2 TABLESPOONS MARGARINE, DIVIDED
    ⅓ CUP SKIM MILK
    3 CUPS DICED RUTABAGA
      SALT* AND PEPPER TO TASTE
    1 TABLESPOON CHOPPED FRESH PARSLEY

Method

1. Peel, dice, and cook potatoes; mash with 1 tablespoon margarine and milk.
2. Preheat oven to 400° F.
3. Put potatoes in 2-quart baking dish, forming a nest in center. Bake for 20 minutes or until lightly browned.
4. While potato is in oven, cook rutabaga until tender. Drain. Season with salt, pepper, and remaining 1 tablespoon margarine.
5. Spoon into potato nest.
6. Sprinkle with chopped parsley.

*Na content of salt not included in estimate.

Baked Acorn Squash with Apple Stuffing

Yield: 2 servings

Exchanges per ½-squash serving:

   1 Bread

   1 Fat

   1 Fruit

Estimated nutrients per serving:

CAL	173	FAT	5
CHO	30	Na	175*
PRO	2	K	606

Ingredients

   1 MEDIUM ACORN SQUASH

   2 SMALL APPLES, UNPEELED, DICED

   2 TABLESPOONS DICED CELERY

   2 TEASPOONS MINCED ONION

   2 TEASPOONS MARGARINE, MELTED

   2 TABLESPOONS WATER

     DASH OF SALT*

Method

1. Preheat oven to 400° F.
2. Cut squash in half. Remove seeds. Place cut side down on baking sheet sprayed with vegetable pan spray.
3. Combine apples, celery, and onion. Add margarine and water. Put in small baking dish. Cover.
4. Bake squash and apple stuffing for 45 minutes or until tender. Remove from oven.
5. Salt squash. Fill with apple mixture.

*Na content of salt not included in estimate.

Winter Squash with Cranberries

Yield: 2 cups
Exchanges per ½-cup serving:
  1 Bread
  1 Fat

Estimated nutrients per serving:

CAL	97	FAT	5
CHO	10	Na	326
PRO	3	K	271

Ingredients

1½ CUPS COOKED, MASHED WINTER SQUASH (OR 1 12-OUNCE PACKAGE FROZEN)
  1 EGG, BEATEN
 ½ CUP COARSELY CHOPPED CRANBERRIES
 ½ TEASPOON SALT
   DASH PEPPER
  1 TABLESPOON MARGARINE, MELTED
   DASH NUTMEG

Method

1. Preheat oven to 400° F.
2. Thaw squash, if frozen. Combine with egg.
3. Stir in cranberries, salt, and pepper.
4. Turn into 1½-quart casserole. Drizzle melted margarine over top. Sprinkle with nutmeg.
5. Bake for 35 to 40 minutes.

Gourmet Golden Squash

Yield: 3 cups

Exchanges per ½-cup serving:

    1 Vegetable

    1 Bread

    1 Fat

Estimated nutrients per serving:

CAL	134	FAT	6
CHO	18	Na	404
PRO	2	K	524

Ingredients

  ½ CUP FINELY CHOPPED ONION

  1 TABLESPOON MARGARINE

  3 CUPS WINTER SQUASH, COOKED AND MASHED
    (OR 2 12-OUNCE FROZEN PACKAGES, THAWED)

  ½ CUP DAIRY SOUR CREAM

  1 TEASPOON SALT

  ¼ TEASPOON PEPPER

    DASH OF NUTMEG

Method

1. Preheat oven to 400° F.
2. Saute onions in margarine until tender.
3. Combine all ingredients. Turn into 1-quart casserole.
4. Sprinkle with nutmeg. Bake uncovered 35 to 45 minutes.

Zucchini and Spinach Casserole

Yield: 3 cups

Exchanges per ½-cup serving:
    1 Medium-Fat Meat
    1 Vegetable

Estimated nutrients per serving:

CAL	102	FAT	6
CHO	4	Na	547
PRO	8	K	250

Ingredients

  1 10-OUNCE PACKAGE FROZEN CHOPPED SPINACH
½ TEASPOON NUTMEG
  2 CUPS SLICED ZUCCHINI
  2 TABLESPOONS WATER
  1 TEASPOON MARGARINE
  1 TEASPOON SEASONED SALT
½ CUP GRATED PARMESAN CHEESE
½ CUP GRATED SWISS CHEESE (ABOUT 2 OUNCES)

Method

1. Preheat oven to 350° F.
2. Cook spinach according to package instructions. Drain; add nutmeg.
3. Combine zucchini, water, margarine, and seasoned salt in skillet. Cover; steam for 5 minutes.
4. Mix Parmesan and Swiss cheeses. In 8-inch casserole, layer spinach, zucchini, and cheese mixture. Bake for 20 minutes.

Cheese-Stuffed Zucchini

Yield: 4 servings
Exchanges per ½-zucchini
serving:

   1 High-Fat Meat
   1 Vegetable
  ½ Bread

Estimated nutrients per serving:

CAL	153	FAT	9
CHO	11	Na	592
PRO	7	K	216

Ingredients

  2 SMALL ZUCCHINI (6–8 INCHES)
 ½ TEASPOON SALT
  2 SLICES BREAD, CRUMBLED
 ½ CUP GRATED PARMESAN CHEESE
    DASH PEPPER
    DASH OREGANO
    DASH GARLIC POWDER
  2 TABLESPOONS MARGARINE, MELTED
    DASH PAPRIKA

Method

1. Trim off ends of zucchini. Cut in half lengthwise.
2. Simmer in boiling salted water until tender, about 5 minutes. Drain. Cool.
3. Scoop out center portion and reserve for filling.
4. Combine reserved pulp with remaining ingredients; mix well. Stuff zucchini with mixture. Sprinkle with paprika.
5. Broil 5 or 6 inches from heat until browned.

Stewed Tomato and Okra

Yield: 3 cups

Exchanges per ½-cup serving:
1 Vegetable
½ Fat

Estimated nutrients per serving:

CAL	42	FAT	2
CHO	5	Na	184
PRO	1	K	184

Ingredients

- 1 10-OUNCE PACKAGE FROZEN OKRA, COOKED
- ¼ CUP CHOPPED ONION
- ¼ CUP CHOPPED GREEN PEPPER
- 2 TEASPOONS VEGETABLE OIL
- ½ TEASPOON SALT
- ¼ TEASPOON PEPPER
- 1 CUP CANNED TOMATOES

Method

1. Cook okra according to package directions. Drain.
2. Cook onion and green pepper in oil until tender.
3. Add seasoning, okra, and tomatoes.
4. Cook on low heat until bubbly.

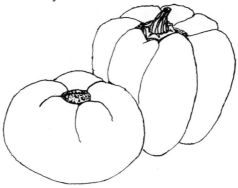

Broiled Tomatoes

Yield: 8 halves (4 servings):   Estimated nutrients per serving:

Exchanges per 2-half serving:

1	Vegetable	CAL	76	FAT	4
1	Fat	CHO	8	Na	318
		PRO	2	K	220

Ingredients

  4 MEDIUM RIPE TOMATOES
¼ CUP CRACKER CRUMBS
½ TEASPOON SALT
    DASH OF PEPPER
  1 TABLESPOON VEGETABLE OIL
    FRESH PARSLEY (OPTIONAL)

Method

1. Wash tomatoes, slice in half crosswise. Place on baking sheet, cut side up.
2. Mix crumbs, seasonings, and oil.
3. Sprinkle 1 tablespoon mixture on each tomato.
4. Broil 8 to 10 inches from heat about 4 minutes or until golden brown. Garnish with parsley sprigs.

Herb-Stuffed Potatoes

Yield: 8 halves (8 servings)

Exchanges per one-half
serving:

    1 Bread
    ½ Fat

Estimated nutrients per serving:

CAL	110	FAT	2
CHO	19	Na	328*
PRO	4	K	470

Ingredients

  4 LARGE BAKING POTATOES (ABOUT 4½ INCHES LONG)
  4 TEASPOONS MARGARINE
  1 5⅓-OUNCE CAN EVAPORATED SKIM MILK
  1 TEASPOON SNIPPED CHIVES
  1 TEASPOON SNIPPED PARSLEY
  ⅛ TEASPOON DRIED SAGE
    SALT* TO TASTE
    PEPPER TO TASTE
    DASH PAPRIKA

Method

1. Preheat oven to 400° F.
2. Bake potatoes about 45 minutes.
3. Cut in half lengthwise. Scoop out inside and mash.
4. Add remaining ingredients except paprika. Mix thoroughly.
5. Spoon potato into shells on baking sheet. Sprinkle with paprika.
6. Return to oven for 10 minutes or until lightly browned.

*Na content of salt not included in estimate.

Speedy Baked Potato

Yield: 8 halves (4 servings)
Exchanges per 2-half serving:
    2 Bread

Estimated nutrients per serving:

CAL	148	FAT	—
CHO	33	Na	6
PRO	4	K	782

Ingredients

  4 LARGE BAKING POTATOES (ABOUT 4½ INCHES LONG)
     PAPRIKA (OPTIONAL)

Method

1. Preheat oven to 400° F.
2. Spray baking pan with vegetable pan spray.
3. Wash and cut potatoes in half lengthwise. Place halves cut side down on pan.
4. Bake about 30 minutes. Sprinkle with paprika, if desired.

Baked Potato and Onion

Yield: 4 servings
Exchanges per 1-potato
serving:
    2 Bread
    1 Fat

Estimated nutrients per serving:

CAL	181	FAT	5
CHO	30	Na	55*
PRO	4	K	822

Ingredients

  4 BAKING POTATOES, PEELED (ABOUT 4½ INCHES LONG)
  4 TEASPOONS MARGARINE, MELTED
  1 MEDIUM ONION, SLICED
    SALT* AND PEPPER AS DESIRED

Method

1. Preheat oven to 400° F.
2. Cut each potato in 4 crosswise slices.
3. Brush margarine between slices and over top.
4. Reassemble potato, with onion slices between potato slices. Hold together with toothpicks. Sprinkle with salt and pepper.
5. Wrap each potato in heavy-duty aluminum foil or double thickness of lightweight foil.
6. Bake on baking sheet 45 minutes or until potatoes are tender.
7. Open foil and return potatoes to oven to brown tops.

*Na content of salt not included in estimate.

Crispy Scalloped Potatoes

Yield: 2 cups
Exchanges per ½-cup serving:

1 Bread	
1 Fat	

Estimated nutrients per serving:

CAL	107	FAT	3
CHO	16	Na	621
PRO	4	K	330

Ingredients

2 CUPS THINLY SLICED RAW POTATOES
1 TABLESPOON FLOUR
1 TABLESPOON MINCED ONION
1 TEASPOON SALT
DASH PEPPER
1 CUP SKIM MILK
1 TABLESPOON MARGARINE

Method

1. Preheat oven to 350° F.
2. Lightly coat 1-quart casserole with vegetable pan spray.
3. Layer half of the potato in bottom of baking dish. Sprinkle with half of flour, onion, salt, and pepper. Repeat layers.
4. Pour milk over the potatoes. Dot with margarine.
5. Cover; bake for 30 minutes.
6. Uncover and bake an additional 35 to 40 minutes or until potatoes are tender.

Mashed Potato Puff

Yield: 6 cups
Exchanges per 1-cup serving:
    1 Medium-Fat Meat
    1 Bread
    ½ Fat

Estimated nutrients per serving:

CAL	169	FAT	9
CHO	13	Na	244
PRO	9	K	329

Ingredients

  4 MEDIUM POTATOES
  ¼ CUP SKIM MILK
  2 TEASPOONS MARGARINE
  ¼ TEASPOON SALT
  3 EGGS, SEPARATED
  ⅓ CUP SKIM MILK
  1 TEASPOON GRATED ONION
  2 TEASPOONS FRESH CHOPPED PARSLEY
    (OR 1 TEASPOON PARSLEY FLAKES)
  ¾ CUP GRATED CHEDDAR CHEESE (ABOUT 3 OUNCES)

Method

1. Preheat oven to 375° F.
2. Peel, quarter, and boil potatoes until tender. Drain and mash with ¼ cup milk, margarine, and salt.
3. Beat egg yolks and ⅓ cup milk. Add to potato with onion, parsley, and cheese. Mix well.
4. Beat egg whites until stiff. Fold into potato. Turn into 1½-quart casserole.
5. Bake for 35 to 40 minutes or until a knife inserted in the center comes out clean. Serve immediately.

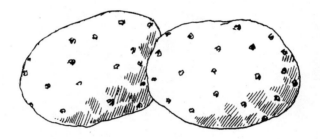

Salads and
Salad Dressings

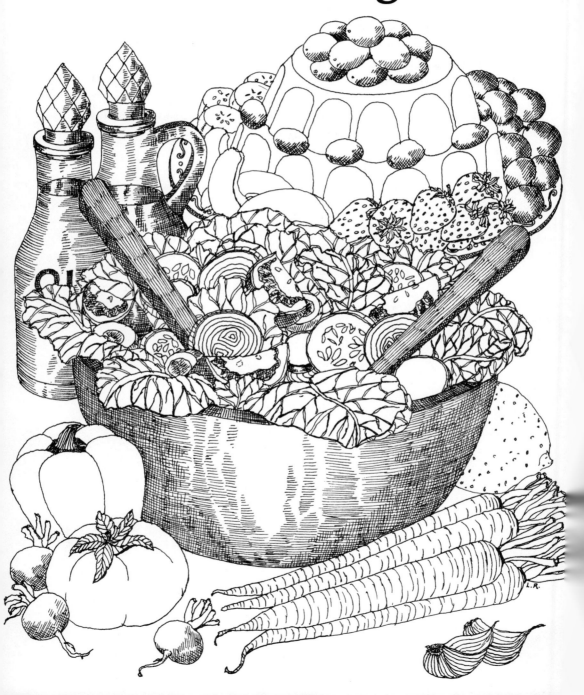

Salads occupy a prominent place on our menus. They may be served as appetizer, side dish, main course, or even as the "finishing touch." Their fresh, chilled ingredients add crispness as well as nutrition to the meal.

The tossed green salad, ever popular, needs no recipe. It can be made differently each time you serve it. Use a variety of greens in place of or in addition to lettuce. Try endive, escarole, romaine, spinach, or other peak-of-the-season greens. Tear greens into fairly large pieces. Add a few other vegetables to suit your mood: cucumber, Chinese cabbage (celery cabbage), radishes, green pepper, raw mushrooms, cauliflower, green onions, bean sprouts, tomatoes. Toss with a light touch and chill until serving time. Use just enough dressing to moisten the greens. Or, for a variety of appetites, serve dressings separately.

The tossed salad becomes a main dish with the addition of strips of chicken, ham, cheese, or hard-cooked egg slices. Another good way to use leftovers!

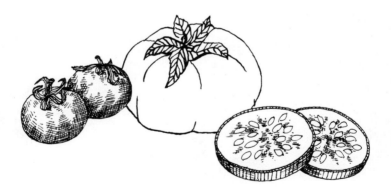

Fruited Chicken Salad

Yield: 4 servings

Exchanges per 1-cup serving:

Estimated nutrients per serving:

CAL	236	FAT	12
CHO	14	Na	388
PRO	18	K	452

- 1 Vegetable
- 2 Lean Meat
- 1 Fat
- 1 Fruit

Ingredients

- 2 CUPS DICED COOKED CHICKEN (8 OUNCES)
- 1 CUP DICED CELERY
- 1 CUP SEEDLESS GRAPES, HALVED
- ½ CUP CANNED UNSWEETENED CRUSHED PINEAPPLE, DRAINED
- 2 TABLESPOONS SLIVERED ALMONDS
- ½ TEASPOON SALT
- ¼ CUP DAIRY SOUR CREAM
- 1 TABLESPOON MAYONNAISE

Method

1. Combine all ingredients. Chill.
2. Serve on lettuce cups.

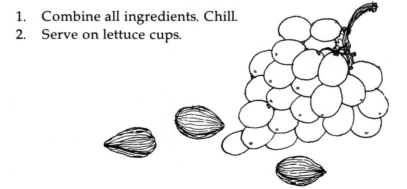

Hot Chicken Salad

Yield: 4½ cups (6 servings)
Exchanges per ¾-cup serving:
    1 Vegetable
    2 Medium-Fat Meat
 1½ Fat

Estimated nutrients per serving:

CAL	263	FAT	19
CHO	7	Na	363
PRO	16	K	369

Ingredients

  2 CUPS DICED COOKED CHICKEN (8 OUNCES)
  2 CUPS CHOPPED CELERY
 ¼ CUP SLIVERED ALMONDS
  2 TABLESPOONS CHOPPED PIMIENTO
 ¼ CUP CHOPPED GREEN PEPPER
 ¼ CUP CHOPPED ONION
 ½ TEASPOON SALT
  2 TABLESPOONS LEMON JUICE
 ⅓ CUP MAYONNAISE
 ¼ CUP GRATED SWISS CHEESE (ABOUT 1 OUNCE)
  2 CUPS COARSELY CRUSHED POTATO CHIPS (2 OUNCES)

Method

1. Preheat oven to 350° F.
2. Mix together all ingredients except cheese and potato chips.
3. Turn into 2-quart casserole.
4. Top with cheese and potato chips.
5. Bake about 25 minutes until cheese is melted.

Mexican Salad Supper

Yield: 10 cups

Exchanges per 1-cup serving:
- 1 Medium-Fat Meat
- ½ Vegetable
- 1 Bread
- 1 Fat

Estimated nutrients per serving:

CAL	207	FAT	11
CHO	17	Na	89
PRO	10	K	381

Ingredients

- ½ POUND GROUND BEEF
- ¼ CUP CHOPPED ONION
- ½ MEDIUM HEAD LETTUCE, SHREDDED
- 2 CUPS TORTILLA CHIPS, COARSELY CRUSHED (ABOUT 4 OUNCES)
- 1 AVOCADO, DICED
- 1 SMALL TOMATO, CHOPPED
- 1 CUP SHREDDED CHEDDAR CHEESE (ABOUT 4 OUNCES)
- 1 1-POUND CAN KIDNEY BEANS

Method

1. Brown ground beef and onion. Drain; chill.
2. Shred lettuce; store in plastic bag in refrigerator.
3. Crush corn chips; set aside.
4. Toss together in large mixing bowl avocado, tomato, cheese, and beans. Chill.
5. At serving time, combine all ingredients.

This salad scarcely needs dressing. Provide French dressing and let your guests add their own amount.

Greek Salad

Yield: 16 cups

Exchanges per 1-cup serving:
- 1 Vegetable
- 1 Fat

Estimated nutrients per serving:

CAL	77	FAT	5
CHO	5	Na	250
PRO	3	K	219

Ingredients

- 1 GARLIC CLOVE
- 1 MEDIUM HEAD LETTUCE, SHREDDED
- 3 MEDIUM TOMATOES, CUT IN EIGHTHS
- 1 MEDIUM CUCUMBER, SLICED
- 6 GREEN ONIONS, SLICED
- 3 STALKS CELERY, DICED
- 1 MEDIUM GREEN PEPPER, DICED
- 6 RADISHES, SLICED
- 1 CARROT, SHREDDED
- 2 TABLESPOONS CHOPPED FRESH PARSLEY
- 1 TEASPOON SALT
- 1/8 TEASPOON PEPPER
- 1/4 CUP OLIVE OIL
- 1 TABLESPOON VINEGAR OR LEMON JUICE
- 1 BEET, CANNED OR COOKED, SLICED
- 4 OUNCES FETA CHEESE, CRUMBLED
- 8 RIPE OLIVES
- 1/4 CUP COOKED CHICK PEAS

Method

1. Rub large salad bowl with garlic.
2. Combine next eleven ingredients.
3. Toss lightly with olive oil. Sprinkle with vinegar. Toss again.
4. Garnish with border of sliced beet and feta cheese.
5. Arrange olives in center and sprinkle chick peas over all.

Marinated Vegetable Buffet

Yield: 5 cups

Exchanges per ½-cup serving:
1 Vegetable
½ Fat

Estimated nutrients per serving:

CAL	51	FAT	3
CHO	5	Na	118
PRO	1	K	160

Ingredients

2 CUPS FRESH CAULIFLOWER (ABOUT ½ of 4-INCH DIAMETER HEAD)
2 CUPS FRESH GREEN BEANS (ABOUT ½ POUND)
¾ CUP SLICED CARROT
½ CUP SLICED ONION
¼ CUP WINE VINEGAR
2 TABLESPOONS SALAD OIL
½ TEASPOON SALT
DILL SEED TO TASTE

Method

1. Separate cauliflower into flowerets. Slice green beans.
2. Cook cauliflower, green beans, and carrots in boiling water 5 minutes. Vegetables should still be crisp. Drain.
3. Add remaining ingredients. Mix well. Refrigerate 6 hours or overnight.

Serving suggestion: Testers felt this Vegetable Buffet could be a snack as well as a salad. Leftovers may be kept in refrigerator for 5 to 7 days.

Spinach Salad

Yield: 4 servings

Exchanges per ¼-recipe serving:

   1 Vegetable

   1 Fat

Estimated nutrients per serving:

CAL	73	FAT	5
CHO	5	Na	67*
PRO	2	K	258

Ingredients

  2 SLICES BACON
  2 CUPS SHREDDED RAW SPINACH
 ¼ CUP CHOPPED GREEN ONION
  1 CUP DICED TOMATO
 ¼ CUP DAIRY SOUR CREAM
   SALT* TO TASTE
   PEPPER TO TASTE

Method

1. Cook, drain, and crumble bacon.
2. Toss all ingredients together.
3. Chill before serving.

*Na content of salt not included in estimate.

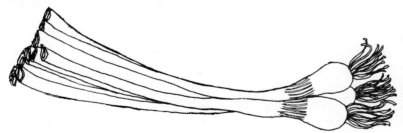

Tabbouli (Wheat Salad)

Yield: 3 cups (6 servings)
Exchanges per ½-cup serving:
    1 Vegetable
    ½ Bread
    1½ Fat

Estimated nutrients per serving:

CAL	131	FAT	7
CHO	15	Na	389
PRO	2	K	186

Ingredients

  ½ CUP FINELY CRUSHED BULGUR
  1 CUP WATER
  1 CUP FINELY CHOPPED FRESH PARSLEY
  ½ CUP CHOPPED ONION
  1 MEDIUM FRESH TOMATO, CHOPPED
  3 TABLESPOONS FRESH LEMON JUICE
  3 TABLESPOONS SALAD OIL
  ½ TEASPOON SALT
  ¼ TEASPOON BLACK PEPPER
    LETTUCE

Method

1. Soak bulgur in water for ½ hour. Drain well.
2. Add vegetables.
3. Mix lemon juice, oil, salt, and pepper. Add to salad. Toss lightly to coat ingredients. Refrigerate for 24 hours.
4. Serve on lettuce leaves.

Tabbouli has as many variations as it does spellings. Try it using 1½ tablespoons each of vinegar and lemon juice in place of 3 tablespoons of juice. For a change add 1 chopped cucumber, or 2 tablespoons fresh mint (1 tablespoon dried mint), or your favorite herbs such as basil or garlic. It keeps so well in the refrigerator that you may prefer to double the recipe.

Two-Bean Salad

Yield: 4 cups (8 servings)
Exchanges per ½-cup serving:
    1 Vegetable

Estimated nutrients per serving:

CAL	39	FAT	1
CHO	8	Na	395
PRO	1	K	114

Ingredients

  1 1-POUND CAN CUT WAX BEANS, DRAINED
  1 1-POUND CAN CUT GREEN BEANS, DRAINED
  ¼ CUP MINCED RED OR YELLOW ONION
  ¼ CUP CHOPPED PIMIENTO
  2 TABLESPOONS FRESH MINCED PARSLEY (OPTIONAL)
3–4 TABLESPOONS CIDER VINEGAR
  ½ TEASPOON SALT
  ½ CUP WATER
    DASH FRESHLY GROUND BLACK PEPPER
  2 TEASPOONS SUGAR

Method

1. Combine beans, onion, pimiento, and parsley.
2. Mix vinegar, salt, water, pepper, and sugar.
3. Toss with beans.
4. Store, covered, in refrigerator overnight or at least 4 hours. Stir occasionally.

Marinated Green Bean Salad

Yield: 3 cups (6 servings)
Exchanges per ½-cup serving:
    1 Vegetable
    ½ Fat

Estimated nutrients per serving:

CAL	55	FAT	3
CHO	5	Na	183
PRO	2	K	106

Ingredients

- ¼ CUP PLAIN LOW-FAT YOGURT
- ¼ CUP DAIRY SOUR CREAM
- ¼ CUP LOW-CALORIE ITALIAN SALAD DRESSING
- 2 MEDIUM TOMATOES, PEELED, CUBED, AND DRAINED
- ½ CUP FINELY CHOPPED ONION
- 1 16-OUNCE CAN CUT GREEN BEANS, DRAINED

Method

1. Mix together yogurt, sour cream, and Italian dressing. Add tomato, onion, and beans; mix well.
2. Chill 3 or 4 hours before serving. Serve in a lettuce cup.

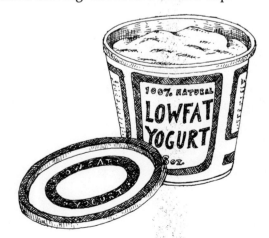

Cauliflower Salad

Yield: 3½ cups (7 servings)
Exchanges per ½-cup serving:
    1 Vegetable
    2 Fat

Estimated nutrients per serving:

CAL	126	FAT	10
CHO	5	Na	274
PRO	4	K	207

Ingredients

  2 CUPS RAW CAULIFLOWER, CUT IN SMALL PIECES
  3 HARD-COOKED EGGS, CHOPPED
  ¼ CUP MINCED ONION
  1 CUP CHOPPED CELERY
  ½ CUP CHOPPED GREEN PEPPER
  1 4-OUNCE CAN PIMIENTO, MINCED
  1 TEASPOON SALT
    PEPPER TO TASTE
  ⅓ CUP MAYONNAISE

Method

1. Cook cauliflower in boiling water 2 minutes.
2. Combine all ingredients.
3. Chill before serving.

Marinated Cucumber

Yield: 2 cups (4 servings)
Exchanges per ½-cup serving:
   1 Vegetable

Estimated nutrients per serving:

CAL	24	FAT	—
CHO	5	Na	141
PRO	1	K	112

Ingredients

- ¼ CUP VINEGAR
- 2 TABLESPOONS WATER
- ¼ TEASPOON SALT
- DASH PAPRIKA
- DASH PEPPER
- 1 MEDIUM CUCUMBER, PEELED AND SLICED
- 1 MEDIUM ONION, SLICED AND SEPARATED INTO RINGS
- 1 TEASPOON MINCED FRESH PARSLEY

Method

1. Combine all ingredients.
2. Chill, stirring occasionally.

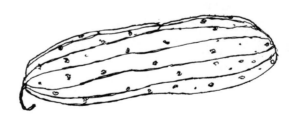

Spicy Cucumber

Yield: 2 cups (8 servings)
Exchanges per ¼-cup serving:
    ½ Vegetable
    ½ Fat

Estimated nutrients per serving:

CAL	39	FAT	3
CHO	2	Na	9
PRO	1	K	57

Ingredients

  1 LARGE CUCUMBER, PEELED AND THINLY SLICED
  1 TEASPOON SALT
  ½ CUP DAIRY SOUR CREAM
  1 TABLESPOON VINEGAR
  2 TABLESPOONS CHOPPED CHIVES
  1 DROP TABASCO SAUCE
  ½ TEASPOON DILL SEED
    DASH PEPPER

Method

1. Slice cucumber into bowl. Sprinkle with salt. Let stand 30 minutes. Drain.
2. Combine rest of ingredients. Mix with cucumbers. Chill before serving.

Easy Coleslaw

Yield: 4 cups (8 servings)
Exchanges per ½-cup serving:
    1 Vegetable
    1 Fat

Estimated nutrients per serving:

CAL	66	FAT	6
CHO	3	Na	187
PRO	1	K	74

Ingredients

3½ CUPS SHREDDED CABBAGE (ABOUT ½ MEDIUM CABBAGE)
¼ CUP SHREDDED CARROTS
¼ CUP CHOPPED GREEN PEPPER
2 TABLESPOONS MINCED ONION
¼ CUP CHOPPED CELERY

Dressing
¼ CUP MAYONNAISE
1 TABLESPOON VINEGAR
2 TEASPOONS SUGAR
½ TEASPOON SALT
½ TEASPOON CELERY SEED

Method

1. Combine all vegetables in a large bowl. Mix well and set aside.
2. Mix together mayonnaise, vinegar, sugar, salt, and celery seed.
3. Pour over vegetables and mix well.
4. Refrigerate until ready to serve.

Wilted Lettuce

Yield: 4 cups
Exchanges per 1-cup serving:
    1 Vegetable
    1½ Fat

Estimated nutrients per serving:

CAL	104	FAT	8
CHO	5	Na	354
PRO	3	K	140

Ingredients

  4 STRIPS BACON
  ½ POUND LEAF LETTUCE
  ¼ CUP VINEGAR
  1 TABLESPOON BACON FAT
  ½ TEASPOON SALT
  ¼ TEASPOON PEPPER
  2 TEASPOONS SUGAR
  2 TABLESPOONS WATER

Method

1. Fry bacon until crisp. Drain, reserving 1 tablespoon of fat; crumble bacon.
2. Shred lettuce into large bowl.
3. Combine remaining ingredients in a skillet. Cook for 2 minutes. Remove from heat.
4. Pour hot vinegar mixture over lettuce and crumbled bacon. Toss until lettuce wilts.

Macaroni Salad

Yield: 4 cups (8 servings)
Exchanges per ½-cup serving:
    1 Bread
    1 Fat

Estimated nutrients per serving:

CAL	114	FAT	6
CHO	13	Na	91
PRO	2	K	104

Ingredients

  1 CUP UNCOOKED ELBOW MACARONI
  ¼ CUP MAYONNAISE
  1 TABLESPOON VINEGAR
  1 TEASPOON PREPARED MUSTARD
  ¾ CUP CHOPPED CELERY
  ½ CUP SLICED GREEN ONION
  2 TABLESPOONS SWEET PICKLE RELISH
  1 TABLESPOON CHOPPED PIMIENTO

Method

1. Cook macaroni; drain.
2. Mix mayonnaise, vinegar, and mustard in large bowl.
3. Add macaroni and remaining ingredients.
4. Chill.

Confetti Potato Salad

Yield: 3 cups (6 servings)
Exchanges per ½-cup serving:
    1 Bread
    2 Fat

Estimated nutrients per serving:

CAL	158	FAT	10
CHO	15	Na	99
PRO	2	K	421

Ingredients

  4 SMALL POTATOES, RAW (ABOUT 1 POUND)
⅓ CUP MAYONNAISE
  1 TEASPOON VINEGAR
  1 TEASPOON PREPARED MUSTARD
¼ CUP DICED CELERY
¼ CUP FROZEN PEAS, COOKED
  2 TABLESPOONS CHOPPED PIMIENTO
    DASH PAPRIKA

Method

1. Cook potatoes in boiling salted water until tender.
2. While potatoes are cooking, mix mayonnaise, vinegar, and mustard.
3. Peel and dice potatoes while hot; add to mayonnaise mixture. Mix well.
4. Fold in celery, peas, and pimiento. Mix well. Top with paprika. Chill 2 to 4 hours before serving.

Red Onion Potato Salad

Yield: 5 cups

Exchanges per ½-cup serving:

1 Bread

Estimated nutrients per serving:

CAL	63	FAT	1
CHO	13	Na	504
PRO	2	K	300

Ingredients

6 MEDIUM POTATOES (ABOUT 2½ INCHES IN DIAMETER)
1 CUP SLICED CELERY
1 CUP THINLY SLICED RED ONIONS
⅓ CUP CHOPPED FRESH PARSLEY
¼ CUP LOW-CALORIE ITALIAN DRESSING
3 TABLESPOONS WINE VINEGAR
2 TEASPOONS SALT
  DASH CAYENNE PEPPER

Method

1. Boil potatoes in skins. Peel and slice while hot.
2. Place potatoes in large bowl. Add Italian dressing; mix well. Chill.
3. Combine remaining ingredients; add to chilled potatoes. Chill until served.

Hot Potato Salad

Yield: 5⅓ cups (8 servings)
Exchanges per ⅔-cup serving:
    1½ Bread
     1 Fat

Estimated nutrients per serving:

CAL	145	FAT	5
CHO	20	Na	472
PRO	5	K	407

Ingredients

  5 MEDIUM POTATOES
  5 SLICES BACON
 ¼ CUP VINEGAR
 ¼ CUP WATER
  1 EGG, SLIGHTLY BEATEN
  1 TEASPOON SUGAR
 ½ TEASPOON SALT
 ¼ TEASPOON PEPPER
 ½ CUP CHOPPED ONION

Method

1. Peel, halve, and boil potatoes. Slice when cool.
2. Cook bacon until crisp. Drain, reserving 1 tablespoon fat. Crumble bacon.
3. In skillet, combine bacon fat, vinegar, water, egg, sugar, salt, and pepper. Heat and stir until thickened.
4. Add potato, onion, and bacon. Mix and heat through.

Carrot Raisin Salad

Yield: 2 cups (4 servings)
Exchanges per ½-cup serving:
    1 Vegetable
    1 Fat
    ½ Fruit

Estimated nutrients per serving:

CAL	101	FAT	5
CHO	13	Na	54
PRO	1	K	273

Ingredients

    2 CUPS SHREDDED RAW CARROT
    ¼ CUP RAISINS
    1 TABLESPOON MAYONNAISE
    3 TABLESPOONS DAIRY SOUR CREAM

Method

1. In mixing bowl combine mayonnaise and sour cream; stir until smooth.
2. Add carrots and raisins. Mix well. Chill.

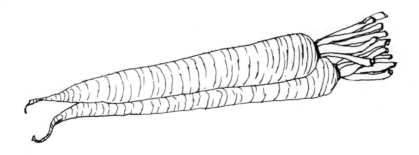

Waldorf Salad

Yield: 4 servings
Exchanges per ¾-cup serving:

    2 Fat

    1 Fruit

Estimated nutrients per serving:

CAL	133	FAT	9
CHO	12	Na	47
PRO	1	K	160

Ingredients

    4 TEASPOONS MAYONNAISE
    2 TEASPOONS UNSWEETENED PINEAPPLE JUICE
    3 SMALL RED APPLES (2½-INCH DIAMETER)
    ½ CUP DICED CELERY
    ¼ CUP CHOPPED WALNUTS

Method

1. Mix mayonnaise and juice.
2. Dice unpeeled apples. Mix with celery and nuts.
3. Fold in dressing.

Variation: If preferred, walnuts may be omitted. Delete one Fat Exchange per serving.

Molded Green Salad

Yield: 3½ cups (7 servings)
Exchanges per ½-cup serving:
   1 Vegetable

Estimated nutrients per serving:

CAL	36	FAT	—
CHO	7	Na	358
PRO	2	K	232

Ingredients

  1 ENVELOPE UNFLAVORED GELATIN
  1 TABLESPOON SUGAR
  1 TEASPOON SALT
1¾ CUPS WATER, DIVIDED
  3 TABLESPOONS VINEGAR
  1 TABLESPOON LEMON JUICE
 ¼ CUP CHOPPED GREEN ONIONS
  2 CUPS SHREDDED RAW SPINACH
  1 CUP CHOPPED CELERY
  1 CUP COARSELY GRATED CARROT (ABOUT 1 CARROT)

Method

1. Combine gelatin, sugar, and salt in saucepan. Add ¾ cup water. Place over low heat, stirring constantly until gelatin is dissolved. Remove from heat.
2. Stir in remaining water, vinegar, and lemon juice.
3. Chill mixture to unbeaten egg white consistency.
4. Fold in remaining ingredients.
5. Turn into a 1-quart mold or 7 individual molds. Chill until firm.

Mandarin Orange Mold

Yield: 4 cups (8 servings)
Exchanges per ½-cup serving:
   1½ Fruit

Estimated nutrients per serving:

CAL	64	FAT	—
CHO	15	Na	NA
PRO	1	K	NA

Ingredients

1 ENVELOPE + 2 TEASPOONS UNFLAVORED GELATIN
1 CUP BOILING WATER
1 6-OUNCE CAN FROZEN ORANGE JUICE CONCENTRATE
1 6-OUNCE CAN COLD WATER
1 11-OUNCE CAN MANDARIN ORANGES IN LIGHT SYRUP, DRAINED

Method

1. Dissolve gelatin in boiling water. Add frozen juice and cold water. Mix well.
2. Divide oranges evenly among molds. Fill with gelatin mixture.
3. Refrigerate. When almost set, stir to distribute orange segments.
4. Chill well to set gelatin firmly.

Serving suggestion: Excellent as a serving of fruit for breakfast.

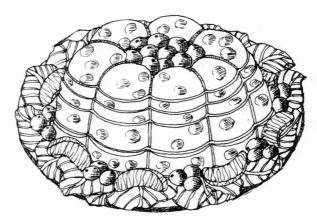

Tangy Apricot Mold

Yield: 4 servings
Exchanges per ¼-recipe serving:

    1 Fruit

Estimated nutrients per serving:

CAL	56	FAT	—
CHO	12	Na	3*
PRO	2	K	308

Ingredients

   1 1-POUND CAN UNSWEETENED APRICOT HALVES
  ½ CUP WATER
   1 ENVELOPE UNFLAVORED GELATIN
      DASH SALT*
   1 TABLESPOON LEMON JUICE
  ½ CUP CLUB SODA

Method

1. Drain and puree apricots in blender or through sieve. (Makes approximately 1 cup of puree.)
2. Combine water, gelatin, and salt in saucepan. Heat to boiling, stirring. Remove from heat.
3. Add lemon juice and apricot puree. Stir to mix well.
4. Add club soda; mix gently.
5. Divide equally into 4 gelatin molds or serving dishes.

*Na content of salt not included in estimate.

Orange Cottage Cheese Mold

Yield: 4 cups (8 servings)
Exchanges per ½-cup serving:
    1 Lean Meat
    1 Fruit

Estimated nutrients per serving:

CAL	78	FAT	2
CHO	9	Na	184
PRO	6	K	159

Ingredients

  1 ENVELOPE UNFLAVORED GELATIN
  ¾ CUP COLD WATER
1½ CUPS ORANGE JUICE
  1 TEASPOON LEMON JUICE (OPTIONAL)
1½ CUPS LOW-FAT COTTAGE CHEESE, SMALL CURD
  ¾ CUP UNSWEETENED CRUSHED PINEAPPLE, DRAINED
  1 TABLESPOON MAYONNAISE

Method

1. Sprinkle gelatin over cold water in saucepan. Place over low heat, stir constantly until gelatin dissolves. Remove from heat.
2. Add other ingredients. Stir until well mixed.
3. Pour into oblong pan or 8 individual molds. Chill until set.

Orange-Apple Pinwheel Salad

Yield: 4 salads
Exchanges per ¼-recipe
serving:
    1 Fruit

Estimated nutrients per serving:

CAL	59	FAT	1
CHO	13	Na	1
PRO	1	K	145

Ingredients

2 ORANGES
2 SMALL APPLES
  LETTUCE

Method

1. Peel and slice oranges.
2. Core and slice apples.
3. Arrange on lettuce with orange and apple wheels alternating.

Variation: 1 grapefruit may be used in place of the 2 oranges. All directions and Exchanges are unchanged.

Creamy Cottage Cheese Dressing

Yield: 1½ cups (8 servings)
Exchanges per 3-tablespoon serving:
   ½ Medium-Fat Meat

Estimated nutrients per serving:

CAL	38	FAT	2
CHO	2	Na	205
PRO	3	K	87

Ingredients

  ½ CUP LOW-FAT COTTAGE CHEESE
  ½ CUP SKIM MILK
  ¼ CUP LEMON JUICE
  ½ TEASPOON SALT
  ½ TEASPOON PAPRIKA
  2 HARD-COOKED EGG YOLKS
  ½ LARGE GREEN PEPPER, QUARTERED
  4 RADISHES, QUARTERED

Method

1. Place all ingredients in blender.
2. Chop only until pepper and radishes are finely chopped, not minced. Refrigerate.

French Dressing

Yield: ¾ cup (6 servings)
Exchanges per 2-tablespoon
serving:
    Free

Estimated nutrients per serving:

CAL	8	FAT	—
CHO	2	Na	132
PRO	—	K	60

Ingredients

  ½ CUP TOMATO JUICE
  2 TABLESPOONS LEMON JUICE OR VINEGAR
  1 TABLESPOON FINELY CHOPPED ONION
  1 TABLESPOON FINELY CHOPPED GREEN PEPPER
  ¼ TEASPOON SALT
  ⅛ TEASPOON BLACK PEPPER

Method

1. Combine all ingredients in jar.
2. Cover and shake well before using.

Garlic Dressing

Yield: 1¼ cups (20 servings)
Exchanges per 1-tablespoon serving:

2 Fat

Estimated nutrients per serving:

CAL	100	FAT	11
CHO	1	Na	141
PRO	—	K	7

Ingredients

- 1 TEASPOON SALT
- ½ TEASPOON PEPPER
- ½ TEASPOON CELERY SALT
- ¼ TEASPOON DRY MUSTARD
- 2 TABLESPOONS WINE VINEGAR
- 2 TABLESPOONS TOMATO JUICE
- ¼ TEASPOON TABASCO SAUCE
- 1 CUP SALAD OIL
- 1 GARLIC CLOVE, PEELED AND CRUSHED

Method

1. Combine ingredients in jar.
2. Cover and shake to blend.

Low-Calorie Blue Cheese Dressing

Yield: 1½ cups (12 servings)
Exchanges per 2-tablespoon
serving:
    ½ Fat

Estimated nutrients per serving:

CAL	25	FAT	1
CHO	1	Na	139
PRO	3	K	29

Ingredients

  1 CUP LOW-FAT COTTAGE CHEESE
  2 TABLESPOONS LEMON JUICE
  ¼ TEASPOON ONION SALT
  ⅓ CUP WATER
  2 OUNCES BLUE CHEESE

Method

1. Put cottage cheese, lemon juice, onion salt, and water into blender.
2. Blend until smooth and creamy.
3. Add blue cheese; blend until nearly smooth.
4. Store in refrigerator. Will keep about 5 days.

Blue Cheese Dressing

Yield: 1½ cups (12 servings)
Exchanges per 2-tablespoon
serving:

    1 Fat

Estimated nutrients per serving:

CAL	46	FAT	4
CHO	1	Na	138
PRO	2	K	40

Ingredients

  4 OUNCES BLUE CHEESE
  ¼ CUP SOUR CREAM
  ¼ CUP SKIM MILK

Method

1. Crumble blue cheese.
2. Add sour cream; stir with fork.
3. Add skim milk and stir until blended.
4. Store in covered jar in refrigerator.

Breads and Sandwiches

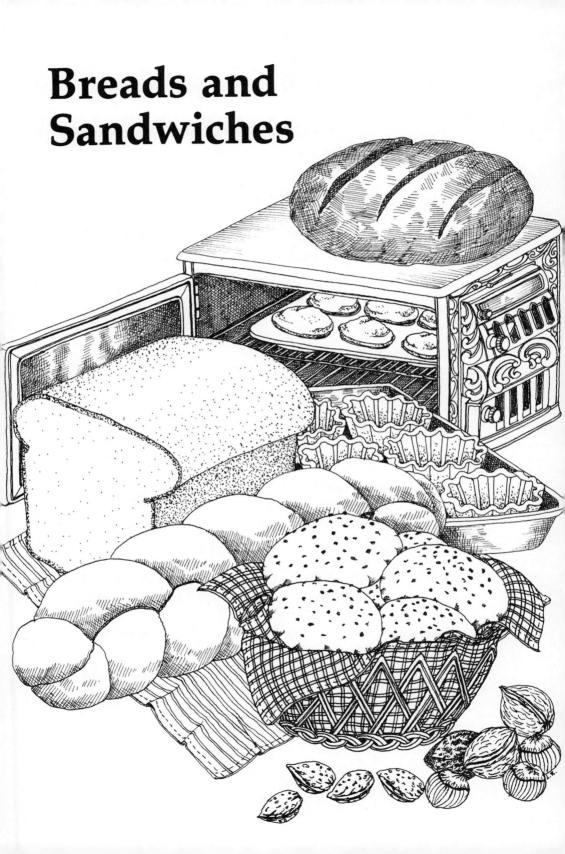

Even a simple meal becomes special when served with a bread warm from the oven. Here you will find biscuits, muffins, popovers, corn bread, fruit and nut breads, and more.

Baking Powder Biscuits

Yield: 12 biscuits

Exchanges per biscuit serving:

    1 Bread

    1 Fat

Estimated nutrients per serving:

CAL	112	FAT	4
CHO	16	Na	291
PRO	3	K	45

Ingredients

  2 CUPS FLOUR
  1 TABLESPOON BAKING POWDER
  1 TEASPOON SALT
  ¼ CUP VEGETABLE SHORTENING
  ¾ CUP SKIM MILK

Method

1. Preheat oven to 450° F.
2. Mix dry ingredients in large bowl.
3. Cut in shortening with pastry blender until mixture resembles coarse crumbs.
4. Add milk; mix quickly.
5. Turn dough onto lightly floured surface. Knead 6 to 8 strokes to mix thoroughly. Roll ½ inch thick, cut with 2-inch biscuit cutter.
6. Place on ungreased baking sheet. Bake 12 to 15 minutes.

Bran Muffins

Yield: 12 muffins

Exchanges per muffin serving:
- 1½ Bread
- ½ Fat

Estimated nutrients per serving:

CAL	123	FAT	3
CHO	20	Na	301
PRO	4	K	191

Ingredients

- 1 EGG
- ¼ CUP SUGAR
- 1¾ CUPS SKIM MILK
- 1½ TABLESPOONS MELTED MARGARINE, COOLED
- 2 CUPS BRAN CEREAL (NOT FLAKES)
- 1 CUP FLOUR
- 1 TABLESPOON BAKING POWDER
- ½ TEASPOON SALT

Method

1. Preheat oven to 400° F.
2. Beat egg; add sugar, milk, and margarine. Beat well.
3. Stir in bran. Allow to stand 1 or 2 minutes.
4. Sift dry ingredients together; add to bran mixture. Stir to blend; do not beat.
5. Spray muffin pan with vegetable pan spray. Fill wells two-thirds full.
6. Bake 25 to 30 minutes, until lightly browned.

Double Corn Muffins

Yield: 12 muffins

Exchanges per muffin serving:

    1½ Bread
      1 Fat

Estimated nutrients per serving:

CAL	150	FAT	6
CHO	20	Na	503
PRO	4	K	91

Ingredients

    1 CUP CORNMEAL
    1 CUP FLOUR
    4 TEASPOONS BAKING POWDER
    1 TABLESPOON SUGAR
    1 TEASPOON SALT
   ¼ CUP VEGETABLE OIL
    1 CUP SKIM MILK
    1 EGG, BEATEN
    1 CUP WHOLE KERNEL CORN, DRAINED

Method

1. Preheat oven to 425° F.
2. Combine dry ingredients.
3. Combine oil, milk, and egg.
4. Add liquid to dry ingredients, mixing only enough to dampen flour. Fold in corn.
5. Spray muffin pan with vegetable pan spray. Fill muffin wells two-thirds full with batter.
6. Bake 20 to 25 minutes.

Surprise Rolls

Yield: 12 rolls
Exchanges per roll serving:
    1 Lean Meat
    1 Bread

Estimated nutrients per serving:
CAL	113	FAT	1
CHO	20	Na	290
PRO	6	K	71

Ingredients

   1 PACKAGE DRY YEAST
  ¼ CUP VERY WARM WATER
   1 CUP LOW-FAT COTTAGE CHEESE, SMALL CURD
   1 TABLESPOON SUGAR
   1 TEASPOON SALT
  ¼ TEASPOON SODA
   1 EGG, BEATEN
2½ CUPS FLOUR, DIVIDED

Method

1. Dissolve yeast in very warm water in large bowl.
2. Warm cottage cheese in saucepan over low heat. Remove from heat.
3. Add cottage cheese, sugar, salt, soda, egg, and ½ cup flour to yeast. Beat at medium speed of electric mixer 2 minutes.
4. Gradually add remaining flour to form a soft dough. Turn out onto floured board. Knead for 10 minutes. Place dough in a greased bowl, turning to grease all sides. Cover and let rise in a warm place free from draft until double in bulk, about 1½ hours.
5. Punch dough down. Turn out onto a floured board; divide dough into 12 equal pieces; shape into balls.
6. Place balls in 9-inch round baking pan sprayed with vegetable pan spray. Cover; let rise in warm place until doubled in bulk, about 30 minutes.
7. Bake at 350° F for 20 minutes.

Matzo Meal Popovers

Yield: 12 popovers
Exchanges per popover serving:

    1 Bread
    1 Fat

Estimated nutrients per serving:

CAL	160	FAT	12
CHO	10	Na	114
PRO	3	K	24

Ingredients

    1 CUP WATER
    ½ CUP VEGETABLE OIL
    1 CUP MATZO MEAL
    ½ TEASPOON SALT
    2 TABLESPOONS SUGAR
    4 EGGS

Method

1. Preheat oven to 400° F.
2. Bring water and oil to a rapid boil. Remove from heat.
3. Add matzo meal, salt, and sugar. Mix well.
4. Add eggs, one at a time, beating after each addition.
5. Coat muffin tins with vegetable pan spray.
6. Fill muffin wells half full with batter.
7. Bake in preheated 400° F oven for 15 minutes; reduce heat to 375° F for 45 minutes.

Scones

Yield: 18 scones
Exchanges per scone serving:
    1 Bread

Estimated nutrients per serving:

CAL	74	FAT	2
CHO	12	Na	219
PRO	2	K	29

Ingredients

  2 CUPS SIFTED FLOUR
  1 TABLESPOON BAKING POWDER
  1 TEASPOON SALT
  2 TABLESPOONS SUGAR
  3 TABLESPOONS MARGARINE
½ CUP SKIM MILK
  1 EGG, SLIGHTLY BEATEN

Method

1. Preheat oven to 450° F.
2. Sift together flour, baking powder, salt, and sugar.
3. Cut in margarine.
4. Stir in milk and egg.
5. Turn dough onto lightly floured board. Roll or pat dough ½ inch thick. Cut into 2-inch rounds.
6. Place on ungreased baking sheet. Bake 10 to 12 minutes, until brown. Serve hot.

Chapatties

Yield: 12 chapatties
Exchanges per chapatty serving:
    1 Bread
    1½ Fat

Estimated nutrients per serving:
CAL 131   FAT 7
CHO 15   Na 208
PRO 2   K 75

Ingredients

  2 CUPS FLOUR
  1 TEASPOON SALT
  ¼ CUP VEGETABLE OIL
  ½ CUP WATER, SCANT
  2 TABLESPOONS MARGARINE, MELTED

Method

1. Sift together flour and salt. Blend in oil using fork or pastry blender.
2. Add water, using hands to mix well. On a floured board knead 5 minutes until dough is shiny.
3. Divide dough into 12 pieces. Roll each to about 5- to 7-inch circle.
4. Brown lightly on hot grill coated with vegetable pan spray.
5. Brush with margarine.

Serving suggestion: Good with Curried Lamb (see index).

Cottage Cheese Breakfast Rolls

Yield: 8 rolls
Exchanges per roll serving:
    ½ Lean Meat
    1 Bread
    1 Fat
    ½ Fruit

Estimated nutrients per serving:
CAL 176   FAT 8
CHO 19   Na NA
PRO 7   K NA

Ingredients

Filling

- 2 EGGS, SLIGHTLY BEATEN
- 2 TABLESPOONS SUGAR
- ¼ TEASPOON CINNAMON
  - DASH NUTMEG
- ⅓ CUP NONFAT DRY MILK POWDER
- ¼ CUP WATER
- 1 CUP 1% LOW-FAT COTTAGE CHEESE, SMALL CURD
- 1 TEASPOON VANILLA

- 1 PACKAGE READY-TO-BAKE REFRIGERATOR CRESCENT ROLLS (8 PER PACKAGE)
- 1 TABLESPOON MELTED MARGARINE
- ½ CUP UNSWEETENED APPLESAUCE

Method

1. Preheat oven to 325° F.
2. Combine all filling ingredients and place in an 8- × 8-inch baking dish coated with vegetable pan spray. Bake for 25 minutes. Let cool.
3. Place crescent rolls on cookie sheet; spread out into thin squares of dough. Brush with melted margarine. Spoon filling equally on rolls. Bring corners of dough together at center. Brush any remaining margarine on top of rolls.
4. Bake according to directions on crescent roll package. Cool.
5. Top each roll with 1 tablespoon applesauce and serve.

Serving suggestion: Excellent for breakfast. If desired, filling can be made in advance to save time in the morning.

Individual Cheese Apple Danish

Yield: 1 serving

Exchanges per serving:
  1 High-Fat Meat
  1 Bread
  1 Fruit

Estimated nutrients per serving:

CAL	208	FAT	8
CHO	25	Na	219
PRO	9	K	148

Ingredients

  1 CUP WATER
  ½ TEASPOON CINNAMON
  DASH NUTMEG
  1 SMALL APPLE, CORED, PEELED, AND THINLY SLICED
  1 SLICE BREAD, TOASTED
  1 1-OUNCE SLICE PROCESSED AMERICAN CHEESE

Method

1. Measure water into small saucepan. Add spices.
2. Add apple slices; bring to a boil. Reduce heat; simmer until apple is tender. Drain.
3. Place apple on toast. Top with cheese.
4. Broil until cheese bubbles.

Basic Crepes

Yield: 24 crepes (12 servings)
Exchanges per 2-crepe serving:
    1 Bread
    1 Fat

Estimated nutrients per serving:

CAL	104	FAT	4
CHO	13	Na	57
PRO	4	K	82

Ingredients

  3 EGGS
⅛ TEASPOON SALT
1½ CUPS FLOUR
1½ CUPS SKIM MILK
  2 TABLESPOONS VEGETABLE OIL

Method

1. In mixing bowl, combine eggs and salt.
2. Add flour alternately with milk, beating until smooth after each addition.
3. Add oil and beat.
4. Refrigerate for at least 1 hour.
5. Cook on upside-down crepe griddle according to manufacturer's directions, or in skillet with nonstick coating. (If using skillet, allow 2 tablespoons batter per crepe, turning skillet to coat evenly in very thin layer. Cook over medium heat until bottom is brown. Turn; brown other side a few seconds.)

Crepes may be made in advance, wrapped in foil or plastic wrap, and stored in refrigerator for 2 or 3 days. For easier separation, a layer of waxed paper or foil may be placed between crepes. They may be kept in freezer if tightly sealed in freezer bags. When ready to use, bring crepes to room temperature before separating. Crepes have many uses. Three recipes appear in this book. One recipe tester reported that her sons liked leftover crepes with applesauce and cinnamon or with peanut butter for breakfast.

Pancakes

Yield: 8 pancakes

Exchanges per pancake serving:

1 Bread

1 Fat

Estimated nutrients per serving:

CAL	120	FAT	4
CHO	17	Na	309
PRO	4	K	79

Ingredients

1¼ CUPS FLOUR

1 TABLESPOON BAKING POWDER

2 TEASPOONS SUGAR

½ TEASPOON SALT

1 EGG, BEATEN

1 CUP SKIM MILK

2 TABLESPOONS VEGETABLE OIL

Method

1. Sift together dry ingredients.
2. Combine egg, milk, and oil. Add to dry ingredients. Stir only until dry ingredients are moistened. (Batter will be lumpy.)
3. Pour ¼ cup batter on hot griddle for each pancake. Turn when pancakes are puffed and bubbly; brown on other side.

Waffles

Yield: 8 waffles

Exchanges per waffle serving:
- ½ Milk
- 1 Bread
- 2 Fat

Estimated nutrients per serving:

CAL	207	FAT	11
CHO	21	Na	322
PRO	6	K	107

Ingredients

- 1¾ CUPS SIFTED FLOUR
- 1 TABLESPOON BAKING POWDER
- ½ TEASPOON SALT
- 2 EGGS, SEPARATED
- 1¼ CUPS SKIM MILK
- ⅓ CUP VEGETABLE OIL

Method

1. Preheat waffle iron.
2. Sift together dry ingredients.
3. Combine egg yolks, milk, and oil. Stir into dry ingredients.
4. Beat egg whites until stiff. Fold into batter.
5. Bake in waffle iron, using scant ½ cup batter per waffle.

French Toast

Yield: 6 slices

Exchanges per 1-slice serving:
- ½ Lean Meat
- 1 Bread
- ½ Fat

Estimated nutrients per serving:

CAL	112	FAT	4
CHO	14	Na	230
PRO	5	K	84

Ingredients

- 2 EGGS, SLIGHTLY BEATEN
- ⅛ TEASPOON SALT
- ½ CUP SKIM MILK
- 1 TABLESPOON MARGARINE
- 6 SLICES DAY-OLD BREAD
  DASH CINNAMON

Method

1. Mix eggs, salt, and milk in pie pan.
2. Melt margarine in skillet.
3. Dip bread quickly in egg mixture to coat.
4. Brown one side in skillet. Sprinkle top side with cinnamon. Turn; brown second side. Serve immediately.

Serving suggestion: Try applesauce or sour cream on French Toast for a change. Remember to count the Exchanges for topping.

Apple Cheese Bread

Yield: 16 ½-inch slices
Exchanges per 1-slice serving:
    1½ Bread
    1½ Fat

Estimated nutrients per serving:

CAL	175	FAT	7
CHO	23	Na	251
PRO	5	K	65

Ingredients

2½ CUPS FLOUR
 ½ CUP SUGAR
 2 TEASPOONS BAKING POWDER
 1 TEASPOON SALT
 ½ TEASPOON CINNAMON
 2 EGGS, BEATEN
 ¾ CUP SKIM MILK
 ¼ CUP VEGETABLE OIL
1½ CUPS SHREDDED CHEDDAR CHEESE (ABOUT 6 OUNCES)
 1 MEDIUM APPLE, DICED (ABOUT 1 CUP)

Method

1. Preheat oven to 350° F.
2. Sift dry ingredients into large bowl.
3. Stir in remaining ingredients in order listed.
4. Pour mixture into 9- × 5-inch loaf pan sprayed with vegetable pan spray.
5. Bake for 1¼ hours or until bread pulls away from the pan.
6. Remove from pan and cool. Let cool thoroughly before slicing.

Applesauce Nut Bread

Yield: 16 ½-inch slices
Exchanges per 1-slice serving:
   1½ Bread
     1 Fruit
     2 Fat

Estimated nutrients per serving:

CAL	231	FAT	11
CHO	30	Na	142
PRO	3	K	138

Ingredients

    1 EGG, SLIGHTLY BEATEN
    1 CUP UNSWEETENED APPLESAUCE
   ½ CUP VEGETABLE OIL
   ½ CUP SUGAR
    1 CUP RAISINS
   ½ CUP CHOPPED WALNUTS
1¾ CUPS FLOUR
    2 TEASPOONS BAKING POWDER
   ½ TEASPOON SALT
1½ TEASPOONS CINNAMON
   ½ TEASPOON GROUND CLOVES

Method

1. Preheat oven to 350° F.
2. Combine first six ingredients and mix well.
3. Sift flour, baking powder, salt, and spices together. Mix into applesauce mixture.
4. Pour into 9- × 5-inch bread pan sprayed with vegetable pan spray.
5. Bake for 1 hour. Cool 10 minutes before removing from pan.

Tip: Let bread cool for several hours or overnight for easier slicing.

Banana Nut Bread

Yield: 24 ⅜-inch slices
Exchanges per 1-slice serving:
    1 Bread
    1 Fat
    ½ Fruit

Estimated nutrients per serving:

CAL	142	FAT	6
CHO	19	Na	104
PRO	3	K	110

Ingredients

- ½ CUP MARGARINE
- ½ CUP SUGAR
- 3 EGGS
- 2¾ CUPS FLOUR, SIFTED
- 1½ TEASPOONS BAKING POWDER
- ½ TEASPOON SODA
- 1 TEASPOON SALT
- 1½ CUPS RIPE BANANAS, MASHED (ABOUT 3 MEDIUM)
- ⅓ CUP CHOPPED WALNUTS

Method

1. Preheat oven to 350° F.
2. Cream together margarine and sugar. Add eggs; beat well.
3. Sift together dry ingredients. Add to eggs alternately with banana, mixing well after each addition. Stir in nuts.
4. Turn into 9- × 5-inch loaf pan coated with vegetable pan spray.
5. Bake 50 to 60 minutes or until done.
6. Remove from pan. Cool on rack.

Cornbread

Yield: 12 servings
Exchanges per 2¼- × 2¼-inch serving:

    1 Bread
    1 Fat

Estimated nutrients per serving:

CAL	125	FAT	5
CHO	16	Na	347
PRO	4	K	75

Ingredients

    1 CUP YELLOW CORNMEAL
    1 CUP SIFTED FLOUR
    1 TABLESPOON BAKING POWDER
    ½ TEASPOON SALT
    ¾ CUP SKIM MILK
    2 EGGS, SLIGHTLY BEATEN
    3 TABLESPOONS VEGETABLE OIL

Method

1. Preheat oven to 425° F.
2. Combine dry ingredients.
3. Add milk, eggs, and oil. Blend well.
4. Pour into 9- × 9-inch baking pan sprayed with vegetable pan spray.
5. Bake for 20 to 25 minutes. Cut into 12 portions. Serve warm.

Cranberry Bread

Yield: 18 ½-inch slices
Exchanges per 1-slice serving:
    1 Bread
    ½ Fat

Estimated nutrients per serving:

CAL	103	FAT	3
CHO	17	Na	102
PRO	2	K	54

Ingredients

   2 CUPS FLOUR
   ½ CUP SUGAR
   ½ TEASPOON BAKING SODA
   ½ TEASPOON SALT
     JUICE AND RIND OF 1 MEDIUM ORANGE
   2 TEASPOONS MELTED MARGARINE
     HOT WATER
   1 EGG, BEATEN
   1 TEASPOON VANILLA
   1 CUP CRANBERRIES, HALVED
   ½ CUP CHOPPED WALNUTS

Method

1. Preheat oven to 350° F.
2. Sift dry ingredients together.
3. Measure together orange juice, grated rind, and melted margarine; add enough hot water to make 1 cup.
4. Stir liquid into dry ingredients. Add remaining ingredients.
5. Cut aluminum foil to fit the bottom of a 9- × 5-inch loaf pan. Spray sides of pan with vegetable pan spray. Add batter.
6. Bake for 1 hour or until toothpick inserted in top of loaf comes out clean.
7. Let stand overnight for easy slicing.

Irish Soda Bread

Yield: 16 wedges
Exchanges per wedge serving:
    1 Bread
    ½ Fat

Estimated nutrients per serving:

CAL	90	FAT	2
CHO	16	Na	303
PRO	2	K	74

Ingredients

  2 CUPS PLUS 2 TABLESPOONS SIFTED FLOUR, DIVIDED
  2 TEASPOONS BAKING SODA
  1 TEASPOON SALT
  2 TEASPOONS SUGAR
  2 TABLESPOONS MARGARINE
  ½ CUP CURRANTS
  1 TABLESPOON GRATED ORANGE RIND
  ½ TABLESPOON CARAWAY SEEDS (OPTIONAL)
  ¼ CUP VINEGAR
  ¾ CUP SKIM MILK

Method

1. Preheat oven to 375° F.
2. Sift together into mixing bowl 2 cups flour, baking soda, salt, and sugar.
3. Cut in margarine with pastry blender until mixture resembles coarse cornmeal. Add currants, orange rind, and caraway seeds. Set aside.
4. Combine vinegar and milk. Add ½ of the liquid to the dry ingredients. Blend quickly. Add remaining liquid and stir only until blended.
5. Turn dough onto floured surface using 2 tablespoons flour. Knead dough 10 times and shape into round loaf. Place in 8-inch round pan sprayed with vegetable pan spray.
6. Bake for 30 to 35 minutes. Remove from oven and cool on wire rack.
7. Cut in wedges to serve.

Onion Cheese Bread

Yield: 8 wedges
Exchanges per wedge serving:
     ½ High-Fat Meat
     1 Bread
     1 Fat

Estimated nutrients per serving:

CAL	174	FAT	10
CHO	15	Na	336
PRO	6	K	102

Ingredients

  ½ CUP CHOPPED ONION
  4 TEASPOONS MARGARINE, MELTED, DIVIDED
1½ CUPS BISCUIT MIX
  1 EGG, BEATEN
  ½ CUP SKIM MILK
  ¾ CUP GRATED CHEDDAR CHEESE (ABOUT 3 OUNCES)
  1 TEASPOON POPPY SEEDS (OPTIONAL)

Method

1. Preheat oven to 400° F.
2. Saute onion in 2 teaspoons margarine until tender.
3. Put biscuit mix in large bowl.
4. Combine egg and milk. Add to biscuit mix.
5. Add onion and half of the cheese. Mix quickly. Spread dough evenly in 8-inch round baking dish sprayed with vegetable pan spray.
6. Sprinkle top with remaining cheese, poppy seeds, and rest of melted margarine.
7. Bake 20 to 25 minutes. Cut in 8 wedges. Serve warm.

Raisin Bread

Yield: 20 slices
   (less than ½ inch thick)
Exchanges per 1-slice serving:
     1 Bread
     1 Fat
     ½ Fruit

Estimated nutrients per serving:

CAL	132	FAT	4
CHO	20	Na	297
PRO	4	K	112

Ingredients

2¾ CUPS SIFTED FLOUR
3½ TEASPOONS BAKING POWDER
 ¼ CUP SUGAR
1½ TEASPOONS SALT
 ⅓ CUP MARGARINE, MELTED
 2 TEASPOONS GRATED ORANGE PEEL
 2 EGGS
1¼ CUPS EVAPORATED SKIM MILK
 ½ CUP RAISINS, CHOPPED

Method

1. Preheat oven to 350° F.
2. Sift dry ingredients.
3. Mix margarine, orange peel, eggs, and milk. Add to dry ingredients. Mix until well blended; stir in raisins.
4. Pour into 9- × 5-inch loaf pan which has been sprayed with vegetable pan spray. Bake 1¼ hours.
5. Remove from pan. Store 12 hours in a cool place before slicing.

Southern Spoon Bread

Yield: 3 cups (6 servings)
Exchanges per ½-cup serving:
    1 Bread
    1 Fat

Estimated nutrients per serving:

CAL	100	FAT	4
CHO	12	Na	314
PRO	4	K	77

Ingredients

  1 CUP BOILING WATER
  ½ CUP CORNMEAL
  ½ CUP SKIM MILK
  ½ TEASPOON SALT
1½ TEASPOONS BAKING POWDER
  1 TABLESPOON VEGETABLE OIL
  2 EGGS, SEPARATED

Method

1. Preheat oven to 375° F.
2. Pour boiling water over cornmeal; stir until smooth.
3. Beat in remaining ingredients, except egg whites.
4. Beat egg whites until stiff; fold into mixture.
5. Turn into 1½-quart casserole sprayed with vegetable pan spray. Bake for 25 to 30 minutes until set.
6. Spoon into serving dishes.

Bread Dressing

Yield: 3 cups (6 servings)
Exchanges per ½-cup serving:
    1 Vegetable
    1 Bread
    1 Fat

Estimated nutrients per serving:

CAL	154	FAT	6
CHO	20	Na	598
PRO	5	K	109

Ingredients

    8 SLICES DAY-OLD OR TOASTED WHITE BREAD
    2 TABLESPOONS MARGARINE
    ¼ CUP CHOPPED ONION
    ½ CUP CHOPPED CELERY
    1 TEASPOON SAGE
    ½ TEASPOON SALT
    ¼ TEASPOON PEPPER
½ to ¾ CUP CHICKEN BROTH
    2 EGGS

Method

1. Preheat oven to 325° F.
2. Cut bread into small cubes. Put in large mixing bowl.
3. Melt margarine in large skillet. Add onion and celery; cook until tender. Add to bread cubes. Add sage, salt, and pepper.
4. Moisten with broth as desired, depending on family preference for dry or moist dressing.
5. Beat eggs lightly with fork. Stir into dressing.
6. Use as stuffing for poultry or other meats, or bake, covered, in 1-quart casserole for 30 minutes.

Fluffy Matzo Balls

Yield: 8 matzo balls
Exchanges per matzo ball
serving:

    ½ Bread
    ½ Fat

Estimated nutrients per serving:

CAL	46	FAT	2
CHO	5	Na	196
PRO	2	K	27

Ingredients

  2 EGGS, SEPARATED
  ½ TEASPOON SALT
    DASH PEPPER
  ½ CUP MATZO MEAL

Method

1. Beat egg whites until stiff. Set aside.
2. Beat yolks until thick and lemon-colored. Add salt and pepper.
3. Using rubber spatula, gently fold egg whites into egg yolks. Add matzo meal gradually. Mix well. Chill dough 5 or 10 minutes.
4. Wet hands with cold water and shape dough into balls, allowing 1 tablespoon per ball.
5. Drop balls, one at a time, into large pot of rapidly boiling water to which 1 tablespoon salt has been added. (Matzo balls puff greatly in size.)
6. Cover; cook about 25 minutes.

To serve: Spoon balls into soup bowls; cover with hot chicken broth.

Garlic Croutons

Yield: 1½ cups (12 servings)
Exchanges per 2-tablespoon serving:
    Free

Estimated nutrients per serving:

CAL	18	FAT	1
CHO	2	Na	75*
PRO	1	K	8

Ingredients

  2 SLICES BREAD
  2 TEASPOONS MARGARINE
     PAPRIKA AS DESIRED
     GARLIC SALT* AS DESIRED

Method

1. Preheat oven to 300° F.
2. Cut bread into ½-inch cubes.
3. Melt margarine in shallow baking pan.
4. Add bread cubes; toss lightly to coat. Sprinkle with paprika and garlic salt.
5. Bake 20 minutes, or until cubes are dry and browned.

Croutons may be stored in an airtight container for salads and soups.

*Na content of garlic salt not included in estimate.

Grilled Cheese Sandwich

Yield: 1 sandwich

Exchanges per serving:

    2 High-Fat Meat

    2 Bread

Estimated nutrients per serving:

CAL	336	FAT	16
CHO	30	Na	1015
PRO	18	K	134

Ingredients

    2 SLICES BREAD

    2 1-OUNCE SLICES SHARP PROCESSED CHEESE

       MUSTARD TO TASTE (OPTIONAL)

Method

1. Make sandwich using 2 slices bread and 2 slices cheese. Spread lightly with mustard if desired.
2. Coat skillet with vegetable pan spray. Brown sandwich on both sides over low heat.

Make as many sandwiches as you wish, using the same proportions and Exchanges. This is a quick lunch—or even breakfast!

Broiled Tuna Burgers

Yield: 8 halves (4 servings)
Exchanges per 2-half serving:

    3 Lean Meat
    ½ Vegetable
    2 Bread
    1 Fat

Estimated nutrients per serving:

CAL	359	FAT	15
CHO	32	Na	1074
PRO	24	K	251

Ingredients

- 1 6½-OUNCE CAN WATER-PACKED TUNA, DRAINED AND FLAKED
- 2 TABLESPOONS CHOPPED ONION
- 2 TABLESPOONS MAYONNAISE
- ½ TEASPOON PREPARED MUSTARD
- 2 MEDIUM TOMATOES, SLICED
- 4 HAMBURGER BUNS (ABOUT 2 OUNCES EACH)
- 4 1-OUNCE SLICES SHARP PROCESSED CHEESE

Method

1. Preheat broiler.
2. Combine tuna, onion, mayonnaise, and mustard. Slice tomatoes in 4 slices each.
3. Split buns; toast.
4. Spoon 2 tablespoons tuna mixture on each half bun. Top with tomato slice and ½ slice cheese.
5. Broil 6 inches from heat 2 or 3 minutes or until cheese melts.

Sloppy Joes

Yield: 3 cups (6 servings)
Exchanges per serving
(scant ½ cup plus 1 bun):
    2 Medium-Fat Meat
    1 Vegetable
    2 Bread

Estimated nutrients per serving:

CAL	316	FAT	12
CHO	34	Na	727
PRO	18	K	547

Ingredients

    1 POUND GROUND BEEF
    ½ CUP CHOPPED ONION
    ½ CUP CHOPPED CELERY
    1 8-OUNCE CAN TOMATO SAUCE
    ½ TEASPOON SALT
      DASH PEPPER
    6 HAMBURGER BUNS (ABOUT 2 OUNCES EACH)

Method

1. Saute ground beef, onion, and celery. Drain excess fat.
2. Add remaining ingredients. Simmer 10 minutes.
3. Spoon onto hamburger buns, allowing scant ½ cup per bun.

Individual Pizzas

Yield: 12 pizzas (6 servings)
Exchanges per 2-slice serving:
    2 Medium-Fat Meat
    1 Vegetable
    2 Bread

Estimated nutrients per serving:

CAL	308	FAT	12
CHO	34	Na	1034
PRO	16	K	425

Ingredients

- ½ POUND GROUND BEEF
- ¼ CUP CHOPPED ONION
- ¼ CUP CHOPPED GREEN PEPPER
- 1 TEASPOON SALT
- 6 ENGLISH MUFFINS, SPLIT
- 2 TABLESPOONS MARGARINE
- 1 8-OUNCE CAN TOMATO SAUCE
- 1 TEASPOON OREGANO
- 1 4-OUNCE CAN MUSHROOM STEMS AND PIECES
- 4 OUNCES MOZZARELLA CHEESE (LOW FAT, PART SKIM), SLICED

Method

1. Preheat oven to 350° F.
2. Brown ground beef with onion, green pepper, and salt. Drain.
3. Split English muffins; spread with margarine. Place on baking sheet.
4. Mix tomato sauce with oregano. Spread on muffin halves (about 1 tablespoon each).
5. Sprinkle on mushrooms. Add meat mixture (about 2 tablespoons).
6. Cover with cheese. Heat about 15 minutes until cheese melts and muffin begins to brown.

Fruits

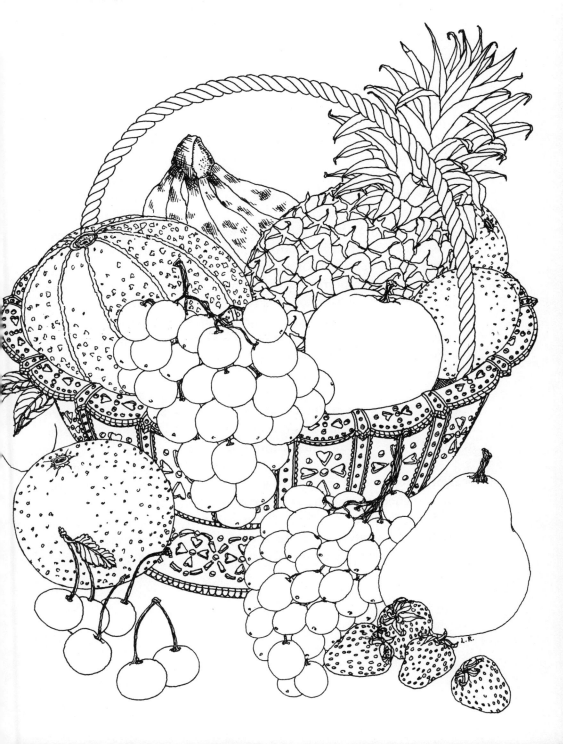

There is nothing more attractive or tempting to most people than a bowl of fresh fruit. For everyone, particularly those who must control carbohydrates and calories, fruit often serves as the perfect ending to a meal.

Fortunately, a panoply of fruits is available year-round. When fresh fruits are gone from the markets, you can rely on canned or frozen varieties processed without sugar. You may want to try canning or freezing your own, using information in another section of this book.

Many companies are now canning fruits in juices. When using the juice-packed fruits, remember to drain the fruit and count the juice as an extra serving.

Fruit cups offer a refreshing way to start—or end—a meal. Almost any favorite fruits can be used for a blend of contrasting flavors and color. A few colorful combinations:

Orange and grapefruit sections with a few pomegranate seeds
Orange sections and sliced banana
Fresh or canned pineapple chunks with strawberries
Melon balls, one or more kinds, with lime or lemon wedges
Sliced peaches and blueberries
Pineapple, banana, and grapes
Canned fruits with unpeeled diced apple or grapes

The possibilities are endless, and you don't need a recipe. To make four servings, for example, combine four Fruit Exchange portions, mix lightly, and divide equally into four serving dishes.

For a special treat, try fruit with cheese. A platter of unpeeled pear or apple wedges dipped in lemon juice to preserve their color, small bunches of grapes, quartered oranges, or other fruits arranged with wedges of a favorite cheese (Brie, Camembert, blue or Roquefort, Muenster, to name a few) and assorted crackers is a pretty centerpiece as well as a delicious way to end a light meal.

Ambrosia

Yield: 2 cups (4 servings)
Exchanges per ½-cup serving:
    ½ Fat
    1 Fruit

Estimated nutrients per serving:

CAL	74	FAT	2
CHO	13	Na	2
PRO	1	K	286

Ingredients

- 2 MEDIUM ORANGES, PEELED AND DICED
- 1 SMALL BANANA, SLICED
- ¼ CUP ORANGE JUICE
- 2 TABLESPOONS SHREDDED COCONUT

Method

1. Combine fruits and juice.
2. Portion in dessert dishes. Sprinkle with coconut.

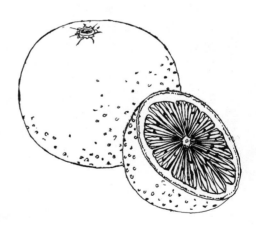

Apple-Pineapple Bake

Yield: 3 cups (6 servings)
Exchanges per ½-cup serving:
    ½ Fat
    1 Fruit

Estimated nutrients per serving:

CAL	66	FAT	2
CHO	12	Na	1
PRO	1	K	86

Ingredients

  3 MEDIUM BAKING APPLES
  ½ CUP UNSWEETENED CRUSHED PINEAPPLE, DRAINED
    (RESERVE JUICE)
  ½ TEASPOON CINNAMON
1½ TEASPOONS SUGAR
  ⅓ CUP RESERVED PINEAPPLE JUICE
  2 TABLESPOONS CHOPPED WALNUTS

Method

1. Preheat oven to 350° F.
2. Peel and slice apples into 8-inch-pie plate sprayed with vegetable pan spray.
3. Spoon pineapple over apples.
4. Sprinkle with cinnamon and sugar.
5. Pour juice over fruit. Sprinkle nuts evenly over top.
6. Bake for 40 minutes. May be served warm or chilled.

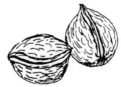

Cherry-Berry Compote

Yield: 4 cups (8 servings)
Exchanges per ½-cup serving:
    1 Fruit

Estimated nutrients per serving:

CAL	53	FAT	1
CHO	12	Na	30*
PRO	1	K	118

Ingredients

    1 1-POUND CAN RED SOUR PITTED CHERRIES
       WATER
    4 TEASPOONS SUGAR
    4 TEASPOONS CORNSTARCH
       DASH SALT*
    2 TEASPOONS LEMON JUICE
    2 CUPS FRESH STRAWBERRIES, QUARTERED

Method

1. Drain cherries; reserve liquid. Add water to make 1½ cups.
2. In saucepan mix sugar, cornstarch, and salt. Stir in liquid. Cook, stirring, until thickened and bubbly.
3. Add lemon juice and cherries. Chill.
4. When cool, add strawberries.

Serving suggestion: Garnish each serving with 1 tablespoon dairy sour cream. Exchange = ½ Fat.

*Na content of salt not included in estimate.

Rosy Apple Rings

Yield: 12 rings (6 servings)

Exchanges per 2-ring serving:

    1½ Fruit

Estimated nutrients per serving:

CAL	73	FAT	1
CHO	17	Na	2
PRO	1	K	132

Ingredients

    1 CUP WATER
    2 TABLESPOONS SEEDLESS RAISINS
    6 SMALL RED APPLES

Method

1. Bring water and raisins to a boil in large skillet. Reduce heat, simmer 10 minutes, stirring occasionally.
2. Wash and core apples. Do not peel. Cut thin slice off top and bottom of each apple; discard.
3. Slice apples in half crosswise to make thick rings. Add to raisin-water mixture and cook slowly 5 to 7 minutes. Turn apples and cook until soft. Do not overcook. (Cooking time will vary with type of apple and thickness of slice.)
4. Serve immediately with raisins sprinkled over apple rings.

Serving suggestion: Use as a garnish on meat platters or dinner plates.

Baked Apples

Yield: 4 servings
Exchanges per apple serving:
    2½ Fruit

Estimated nutrients per serving:

CAL	111	FAT	1
CHO	26	Na	3
PRO	1	K	255

Ingredients

   4 MEDIUM BAKING APPLES (ABOUT 2¾ INCHES DIAMETER)
  ¼ CUP RAISINS
  ½ CUP APPLE JUICE

Method

1. Preheat oven to 375° F.
2. Wash and core apples. Pare a strip from the top of each apple and discard. Place apples in a baking pan.
3. Put 1 tablespoon of raisins in each apple.
4. Pour apple juice over the apples.
5. Bake for 40 minutes, or until done. Baste apples with juice twice during cooking.
6. Serve warm or chilled.

Chunky French Applesauce

Yield: 2 cups (4 servings)
Exchanges per scant ½-cup serving:

    1 Fruit

Estimated nutrients per serving:

CAL	52	FAT	—
CHO	13	Na	2
PRO	—	K	155

Ingredients

  4 MEDIUM COOKING APPLES
  ½ CUP WATER
  1 TEASPOON CINNAMON

Method

1. Peel, core, and slice apples into saucepan. Add water.
2. Simmer, covered, until tender.
3. Add cinnamon.
4. Serve warm or chilled.

Variation: Cooked apple may be put through a food mill or sieved, if smooth texture is desired.

Fruit Compote

Yield: 2 cups (4 servings)
Exchanges per ½-cup serving:

    2 Fruit

Estimated nutrients per serving:

CAL	97	FAT	1
CHO	22	Na	NA
PRO	1	K	NA

Ingredients

  1 1-POUND CAN UNSWEETENED PINEAPPLE CHUNKS, DRAINED
  1 1-POUND CAN UNSWEETENED PEACH SLICES, DRAINED
  2 TEASPOONS GRATED ORANGE RIND
  1 TABLESPOON SHREDDED COCONUT

Method

1. Preheat oven to 400° F.
2. Arrange fruits in baking dish.
3. Sprinkle with orange rind and coconut.
4. Bake 10 or 15 minutes or until hot. Serve warm.

Broiled Grapefruit

Yield: 2 servings
Exchanges per half-grapefruit
serving:

   1 Fruit

Estimated nutrients per serving:

CAL	42	FAT	—
CHO	10	Na	117*
PRO	1	K	132

Ingredients

  1 GRAPEFRUIT
    DASH SALT*
 ⅛ TEASPOON GROUND NUTMEG

Method

1. Cut grapefruit in half crosswise. Remove seeds. With kitchen shears snip out core. Cut around each segment.
2. Sprinkle with salt and nutmeg.
3. Broil on shallow baking pan 4 inches from heat for 5 minutes.

*Na content of salt not included in estimate.

Spiced Peaches

Yield: varies with number of
  peach halves in can

Exchanges per 2-medium-half
  serving:
     1 Fruit

Estimated nutrients per serving:

CAL	40	FAT	—
CHO	10	Na	4
PRO	—	K	234

Ingredients

    1 1-POUND CAN UNSWEETENED PEACH HALVES,
      UNDRAINED
    1 6-INCH CINNAMON STICK
    3 WHOLE CLOVES

Method

1. Pour peaches with their liquid into saucepan. Liquid should cover the fruit.
2. Add cinnamon stick and cloves. Bring to a boil. Reduce heat and simmer 10 minutes.
3. Serve hot or chill in refrigerator and serve as a cold garnish.

Serving suggestions:

1. Serve as a garnish with beef.
2. Place peach halves on lettuce leaf and add ¼ cup low-fat cottage cheese (1 Meat Exchange).

Finishing Touches

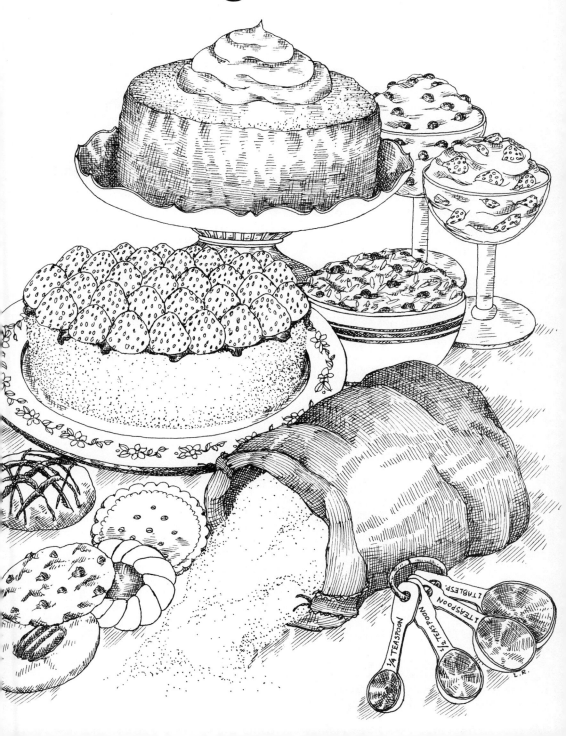

The final satisfying note on a menu may be a dish of fruit. After a light meal you may want a heartier "finishing touch," a smooth creamy custard, a fruit pudding, or on Very Special Occasions something like Strawberry Cheesecake or Sponge Cake with Cocoa Whipped Topping.

You read in the introductory pages of this book that a small amount of sugar has been used in some of the recipes. Measure the sugar carefully, as you do all other ingredients. It has been calculated into the Exchanges listed for each recipe.

Yogurt offers a nutritious alternative for dessert. Yogurts that are sold fruited and flavored have been sweetened, but an 8-ounce carton of plain unflavored yogurt is only a Milk Exchange. Add your own favorite fruit or flavor. Be sure to read the label to determine whether your brand is made from skim, low-fat, or whole milk.

Two yogurt recipes in this section can be prepared without special equipment. The recipe for Plain Yogurt has approximately the same food value as commercially made plain low-fat yogurt. The other is a richer blend which you may want to try when you want a smaller serving.

When using yogurt in any recipe in this book be sure to use the Plain Yogurt recipe or buy it unfruited and unflavored.

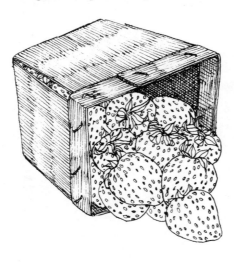

Apricot Sherbet

Yield: 3 cups (6 servings)
Exchanges per ½-cup serving:
2 Fruit

Estimated nutrients per serving:

CAL	72	FAT	—
CHO	16	Na	21
PRO	2	K	242

Ingredients

   1 1-POUND CAN UNSWEETENED APRICOTS
   ⅓ CUP APRICOT NECTAR
   3 TABLESPOONS SUGAR, DIVIDED
   2 TEASPOONS LEMON JUICE
   ⅛ TEASPOON GROUND GINGER (OPTIONAL)
   2 EGG WHITES

Method

1. Drain apricots.
2. Put apricots in blender with nectar, 1 tablespoon sugar, lemon juice, and ginger. Blend until smooth and sugar is dissolved.
3. Pour into small loaf pan. Place in freezer until partially frozen.
4. Beat egg whites until foamy. Add 2 tablespoons sugar and continue beating until egg whites form stiff peaks.
5. In large bowl, beat apricot mixture until smooth. Fold in egg whites. Turn mixture into loaf pan. Cover with foil. Freeze 6 hours or overnight.

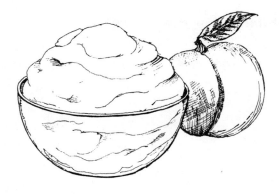

Apricot Whip

Yield: 2½ cups (5 servings)
Exchanges per ½-cup serving:
    1 Fruit

Estimated nutrients per serving:

CAL	56	FAT	—
CHO	12	Na	57
PRO	2	K	165

Ingredients

- ¾ CUP UNSWEETENED CANNED APRICOTS, DRAINED
- 1 CUP PINEAPPLE JUICE, DIVIDED
- 1 ENVELOPE UNFLAVORED GELATIN
- 1 TABLESPOON SUGAR
- ⅛ TEASPOON SALT

Method

1. Puree apricots with ½ cup pineapple juice in blender.
2. Combine gelatin, sugar, and salt in small saucepan. Add remaining ½ cup of juice. Place over low heat, stirring constantly, until gelatin is dissolved. Remove from heat.
3. Stir in pureed apricots.
4. Pour into bowl. Chill until slightly thicker than unbeaten egg white.
5. Beat with electric or hand beater until double in volume.
6. Spoon into dessert dishes. Chill until firm.

Variation: Substitute orange juice for part or all of pineapple juice.

Apple Dumplings

Yield: 8 dumplings
Exchanges per 1-dumpling
serving:

    1 Bread
    1 Fat

Estimated nutrients per serving:

CAL	130	FAT	6
CHO	17	Na	NA
PRO	2	K	NA

Ingredients

  1 PACKAGE READY-TO-BAKE CRESCENT ROLLS (8 IN A PACKAGE)
  4 TEASPOONS SUGAR
  3 TEASPOONS CINNAMON, DIVIDED
  2 SMALL TART APPLES, PEELED AND SLICED
½ CUP WATER
  2 TEASPOONS MARGARINE

Method

1. Preheat oven to 350° F.
2. Separate crescent rolls into 8 pieces. Flatten and stretch each piece.
3. Mix sugar and 2 teaspoons cinnamon. Roll apple slices in this mixture; divide evenly among the rolls. Fold dough over apples and pinch to close openings. Place in baking dish.
4. Mix water, 1 teaspoon cinnamon, and any leftover sugar-cinnamon mixture. Pour over dumplings.
5. Dot each dumpling with margarine.
6. Bake, uncovered, 25 to 30 minutes until rolls are browned.

Apple Rice Pudding

Yield: 4 cups (8 servings)
Exchanges per ½-cup serving:

    1 Bread
    1 Fat
    1 Fruit

Estimated nutrients per serving:

CAL	140	FAT	4
CHO	22	Na	324
PRO	4	K	187

Ingredients

  3 SMALL APPLES, PEELED, CORED, AND FINELY DICED
1½ CUPS COOKED RICE
  1 CUP SKIM MILK
  8 DATES, FINELY SLICED
  1 TABLESPOON SUGAR
 ½ TEASPOON SALT
 ¼ TEASPOON NUTMEG
  1 TEASPOON VANILLA
  1 TABLESPOON VEGETABLE OIL
  3 EGGS, SEPARATED

Method

1. Preheat oven to 325° F.
2. In large bowl stir together all ingredients except egg whites.
3. Beat egg whites until stiff. Fold into apple-rice mixture. Turn into a 1½-quart casserole.
4. Set casserole in a larger baking pan. Set on oven rack. Pour boiling water into larger pan to a depth of 1 inch.
5. Bake for 70 minutes. Serve warm or chilled.

Blueberry Pudding

Yield: 3 cups (8 servings)
Exchanges per ⅜-cup serving:
    ½ Bread
    1 Fat
    1 Fruit

Estimated nutrients per serving:

CAL	121	FAT	5
CHO	18	Na	122
PRO	1	K	63

Ingredients

    1 CUP GRAHAM CRACKER CRUMBS
    2 TABLESPOONS SUGAR
  ½ TEASPOON CINNAMON
    2 TABLESPOONS MARGARINE
    2 CUPS FRESH BLUEBERRIES

Method

1. Preheat oven to 350° F.
2. Combine crumbs, sugar, and cinnamon.
3. Cut in margarine.
4. Place 1 cup berries in a 10- × 6-inch baking dish. Cover with half of crumb mixture. Repeat layers.
5. Bake 30 minutes.
6. Serve warm.

Variation: Use 2 cups fresh sliced peaches in place of blueberries.

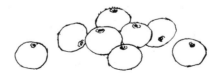

Bread Pudding with Raisins

Yield: 3 cups (6 servings)
Exchanges per ½-cup serving:
　　½ Milk
　　½ Bread
　　½ Fat
　　1 Fruit

Estimated nutrients per serving:
　　CAL 151　　FAT 3
　　CHO 25　　Na 221
　　PRO 6　　K 269

Ingredients

　　3 SLICES DAY-OLD BREAD, CUBED
　½ CUP RAISINS
　　2 CUPS SKIM MILK
　　2 EGGS, SLIGHTLY BEATEN
　　2 TABLESPOONS SUGAR
　　1 TEASPOON CINNAMON
　　1 TEASPOON VANILLA
　¼ TEASPOON SALT

Method

1. Preheat oven to 350° F.
2. Mix bread cubes and raisins in 1½-quart baking dish.
3. Combine remaining ingredients. Pour over bread and raisins; stir.
4. Set dish in shallow pan on oven rack. Pour hot water in pan to depth of 1 inch.
5. Bake 45 to 55 minutes or until knife inserted in pudding comes out clean.

Cherry Crisp

Yield: 3 cups (6 servings)
Exchanges per ½-cup serving:
    ½ Bread
    1 Fat
    1 Fruit

Estimated nutrients per serving:

CAL	108	FAT	4
CHO	16	Na	25
PRO	2	K	115

Ingredients

Fruit layer
  1 16-OUNCE CAN RED SOUR PITTED CHERRIES
1½ TABLESPOONS CORNSTARCH
  4 TEASPOONS SUGAR
  ¼ TEASPOON ALMOND EXTRACT

Topping
  ½ CUP QUICK-COOKING ROLLED OATS
  2 TABLESPOONS CHOPPED WALNUTS
  1 TABLESPOON MARGARINE, MELTED

Method

Fruit layer
1. Drain cherries, reserving ¾ cup juice. Combine small amount of juice, cornstarch, and sugar in saucepan. Stir in remaining juice. Cook over moderate heat, stirring constantly until thickened and clear.
2. Remove from heat. Add cherries and extract.
3. Spread in 8-inch pan.

Topping
1. Preheat oven to 375° F.
2. Mix oats and walnuts in small bowl. Add margarine; mix well with fork. Mixture will be crumbly.
3. Sprinkle topping over cherries.
4. Bake for 20 minutes or until topping is browned.
5. Serve warm or chilled.

Orange Tapioca

Yield: 2 cups (6 servings)
Exchanges per ½-cup serving:

   ¾   Milk
   ½   Fat
   1   Fruit

Estimated nutrients per serving:

CAL	114	FAT	2
CHO	18	Na	66*
PRO	6	K	277

Ingredients

  1½   CUPS SKIM MILK
   1   EGG, BEATEN
   1   TABLESPOON SUGAR
    DASH SALT*
   3   TABLESPOONS QUICK-COOKING TAPIOCA
   ½   CUP ORANGE JUICE
   ½   TEASPOON VANILLA
   ½   CUP DICED FRESH ORANGE

Method

1. Combine milk, egg, sugar, salt, and tapioca in saucepan. Cook on medium heat, stirring constantly, until mixture boils.
2. Remove from heat. Add orange juice slowly, stirring constantly. Return to heat, stirring until mixture boils. Remove from heat.
3. Let cool, stirring occasionally. Mix in vanilla and diced oranges. Chill before serving.

Variation: ½ cup unsweetened peaches, drained and diced, may be used in place of oranges.

*Na content of salt not included in estimate.

Date Tapioca

Yield: 2 cups (4 servings)
Exchanges per ½-cup serving:
 ½ Milk
 1 Bread
 ½ Fat
 1 Fruit

Estimated nutrients per serving:

CAL	162	FAT	2
CHO	30	Na	150
PRO	6	K	407

Ingredients

 1 EGG, SEPARATED
 2 CUPS SKIM MILK
 3 TABLESPOONS TAPIOCA
 ⅛ TEASPOON SALT
 12 DATES, QUARTERED
 ¾ TEASPOON VANILLA

Method

1. Beat egg yolk; mix in saucepan with milk, tapioca, and salt.
2. Let stand 5 minutes.
3. Beat egg white until stiff. Set aside.
4. Bring tapioca mixture to a boil over medium heat. Add dates and cook, stirring constantly, 6 to 8 minutes or until thick.
5. Remove from heat; add vanilla.
6. Gently fold tapioca mixture into egg white.
7. Cool at room temperature, stirring occasionally. Refrigerate until chilled.

Strawberry Cheesecake

Yield: 8 wedges

Exchanges per wedge serving:
1 Lean Meat
½ Bread
½ Fruit

Estimated nutrients per serving:

CAL	128	FAT	4
CHO	15	Na	257
PRO	8	K	169

Ingredients

  2 TABLESPOONS MARGARINE
½ CUP GRAHAM CRACKER CRUMBS
  8 OUNCES LOW-FAT COTTAGE CHEESE
⅓ CUP EVAPORATED SKIM MILK
  2 ENVELOPES UNFLAVORED GELATIN, DIVIDED*
  2 TABLESPOONS SUGAR, DIVIDED
½ CUP ORANGE JUICE
½ TEASPOON GRATED ORANGE RIND
  2 EGG WHITES
⅛ TEASPOON SALT
  2 TABLESPOONS WATER
  1 CUP FRESH STRAWBERRIES, CRUSHED, OR
    UNSWEETENED FROZEN

Method

1. Preheat oven to 400° F.
2. Melt margarine in 9-inch cake pan. Add crumbs, mix. Press mixture over bottom of pan. Bake 5 to 7 minutes. Cool.
3. Sieve cottage cheese or puree in blender. Add milk and stir until smooth. Chill.
4. In saucepan, mix 1½ envelopes gelatin and 1 tablespoon sugar. Add juice and rind. Heat over low heat, stirring constantly until gelatin is dissolved. Remove from heat. Let stand at room temperature.
5. In medium bowl beat egg whites with salt until stiff.

*1 envelope of gelatin equals 1 tablespoon; ½ equals 1½ teaspoons.

6. Fold in gelatin and cottage cheese. Pour over crumbs. Refrigerate until set before adding glaze.

Glaze

1. Mix remaining gelatin (½ envelope) with water and 1 tablespoon sugar. Heat until gelatin is dissolved. Stir in strawberries.
2. Pour mixture over cheesecake and spread with spatula.
3. Refrigerate until firm.

Pineapple Snow

Yield: 6 cups (8 servings)
Exchanges per ¾-cup serving:
    1 Fruit

Estimated nutrients per serving:

CAL	44	FAT	—
CHO	9	Na	51
PRO	2	K	82

Ingredients

  1 ENVELOPE UNFLAVORED GELATIN
  2 TABLESPOONS SUGAR
  ⅛ TEASPOON SALT
  ½ CUP WATER
1½ CUPS UNSWEETENED PINEAPPLE JUICE
  2 EGG WHITES

Method

1. Combine gelatin, sugar, and salt in saucepan. Add water. Place over low heat, stirring constantly until gelatin is dissolved. Remove from heat.
2. Stir in pineapple juice.
3. Chill until mixture begins to thicken.
4. Add egg whites and beat with electric beater until mixture begins to hold its shape.
5. Spoon into dessert dishes. Chill until firm.
6. Serve plain or with soft Custard Sauce (see index).

Strawberry-Pineapple Parfait

Yield: 2 cups (4 servings)
Exchanges per ½-cup serving:
    ½ Bread
    ½ Fat
    ½ Fruit

Estimated nutrients per serving:

CAL	82	FAT	2
CHO	13	Na	29
PRO	3	K	157

Ingredients

  1 ENVELOPE UNFLAVORED GELATIN
  ⅓ CUP COLD WATER
  1 CUP VANILLA ICE MILK
  ½ CUP UNSWEETENED CRUSHED PINEAPPLE, DRAINED
  ¾ CUP UNSWEETENED FROZEN STRAWBERRIES, THAWED

Method

1. Sprinkle gelatin over cold water. Place over low heat, stirring constantly until gelatin dissolves.
2. Add ice milk and fruits. Stir gently until mixed.
3. Portion into 4 individual dishes. Refrigerate until serving time. Do not freeze.

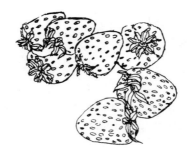

Strawberry Shortcake

Yield: 8 servings
Exchanges per serving
(½-cup berries over 1 biscuit):

    1 Bread
    1 Fat
    1 Fruit

Estimated nutrients per serving:

CAL	157	FAT	5
CHO	25	Na	292
PRO	3	K	161

Ingredients

    1 QUART FRESH STRAWBERRIES
    2 TABLESPOONS SUGAR
    1 TABLESPOON WATER
    8 BAKING POWDER BISCUITS, 2-INCH DIAMETER (SEE INDEX)

Method

1. Wash, drain, and hull strawberries; cut in halves or quarters. Add sugar and water. Refrigerate 2 hours.
2. Split biscuits. Allowing ½ cup of berries per serving, layer half (¼ cup) of berries over bottom of biscuit. Replace top and add remaining berries.

Suggested toppings: 2 tablespoons sour cream or 2 tablespoons whipped cream (without sugar) = 1 additional Fat Exchange, or 1 tablespoon plain yogurt = free.

Raisin Rice Pudding

Yield: 4 cups (8 servings)
Exchanges per ½-cup serving:
   ½ Milk
   ½ Bread
   ½ Fat
   1 Fruit

Estimated nutrients per serving:

CAL	138	FAT	2
CHO	26	Na	303
PRO	4	K	181

Ingredients

   2 EGGS, SLIGHTLY BEATEN
   2 CUPS COOKED RICE
1½ CUPS SKIM MILK
   2 TABLESPOONS SUGAR
   ½ CUP RAISINS
   1 TEASPOON VANILLA
   ½ TEASPOON CINNAMON OR NUTMEG
   ¼ TEASPOON SALT

Method

1. Preheat oven to 350° F.
2. Combine all ingredients.
3. Set a 1½-quart baking dish in shallow pan on oven rack. Pour water to 1-inch depth around dish. Pour pudding in baking dish.
4. Bake for 45 minutes or until knife inserted in pudding comes out clean.

Strawberry Yogurt Mold

Yield: 4 cups (8 servings)
Exchanges per ½-cup serving:
    ½ Fat
    1 Fruit

Estimated nutrients per serving:

CAL	78	FAT	2
CHO	12	Na	NA
PRO	3	K	NA

Ingredients

   1 ENVELOPE UNFLAVORED GELATIN
   2 TABLESPOONS WATER
  ½ 6-OUNCE CAN FROZEN HAWAIIAN PUNCH CONCENTRATE (ABOUT 3 OUNCES)
1½ CUPS FRESH OR UNSWEETENED FROZEN STRAWBERRIES
   1 8-OUNCE CARTON PLAIN LOW-FAT YOGURT
  ¼ CUP DAIRY SOUR CREAM
   2 EGG WHITES
   1 TABLESPOON SUGAR

Method

1. Sprinkle gelatin over water in custard cup. Place in pan of hot water, heat until dissolved.
2. Puree strawberries with punch in blender.
3. Stir in yogurt, sour cream, and dissolved gelatin. Refrigerate until partially set.
4. Beat egg whites with sugar until stiff. Fold into yogurt mixture. Turn into serving bowl or 8 individual dishes. Freeze or refrigerate until set.

Baked Custard

Yield: 3 cups (6 servings)
Exchanges per ½-cup serving:
    ½ Milk
    ½ Medium-Fat Meat

Estimated nutrients per serving:

CAL	83	FAT	3
CHO	8	Na	169
PRO	6	K	171

Ingredients

   3 EGGS, SLIGHTLY BEATEN
   2 TABLESPOONS SUGAR
  ¼ TEASPOON SALT
  ⅛ TEASPOON NUTMEG
   2 CUPS SKIM MILK
  ½ TEASPOON VANILLA
    DASH CINNAMON

Method

1. Preheat oven to 325° F.
2. Combine eggs, sugar, salt, and nutmeg. Slowly stir in milk and vanilla.
3. Set 6 5-ounce custard cups in shallow pan. Pour hot water in pan to level of about 1 inch.
4. Pour custard into cups. Sprinkle with cinnamon.
5. Bake for 40 minutes or until knife inserted in custard comes out clean.

Soft Custard Sauce

Yield: 2 cups (8 servings)
Exchanges per ¼-cup serving:
    ½ Milk
    ½ Fat

Estimated nutrients per serving:

CAL	54	FAT	2
CHO	6	Na	110
PRO	3	K	94

Ingredients

  2 EGGS, SLIGHTLY BEATEN
  2 TABLESPOONS SUGAR
  ¼ TEASPOON SALT
1½ CUPS SKIM MILK
  1 TEASPOON VANILLA

Method

1. Combine all ingredients except vanilla.
2. Cook in double boiler over hot, not boiling, water, stirring constantly. When custard coats a silver spoon, remove from heat.
3. Cool at once by placing pan in bowl of ice water. Stir in vanilla.

Serving suggestion: Serve over fruit (sliced peaches, oranges, banana) or gelatin.

Whipped Topping

Yield: 2 cups (16 servings)
Exchanges per 2-tablespoon serving:

Free

Estimated nutrients per serving:

CAL	12	FAT	—
CHO	2	Na	20
PRO	1	K	67

Ingredients

½ CUP INSTANT NONFAT DRY MILK
½ CUP ICE WATER
2 TEASPOONS SUGAR
½ TEASPOON VANILLA

Method

1. Chill small bowl and beaters.
2. Combine milk powder with ice water in bowl.
3. Beat until stiff.
4. Add sugar and vanilla. Serve immediately.

Whipped Topping may be served on puddings or fruits. It should be used immediately.

Sponge Cake

Yield: 24 slices
Exchanges per slice:
½ Bread
½ Fat
1 Fruit

Estimated nutrients per serving:

CAL	98	FAT	2
CHO	18	Na	43
PRO	2	K	33

Ingredients

  6 EGGS, SEPARATED
  ½ CUP COLD SKIM MILK
1½ CUPS SUGAR
  ½ TEASPOON VANILLA
  ½ TEASPOON LEMON EXTRACT
1½ CUPS SIFTED CAKE FLOUR
  ¼ TEASPOON SALT
  ½ TEASPOON CREAM OF TARTAR

Method

1. Preheat oven to 325° F.
2. Beat egg yolks until thick and light.
3. Add milk gradually, beating until thick. Beat in sugar gradually. Add vanilla and lemon extract.
4. Sift flour with salt. Fold into egg yolk mixture in 4 different portions.
5. Beat egg whites until foamy. Add cream of tartar and beat until stiff. Fold into egg yolk mixture.
6. Bake in ungreased 10-inch tube pan for 1 hour or until top springs back when touched lightly.

Variations:

1. Use one-half recipe. Bake in 9- × 5-inch loaf pan at 325° for 40 minutes. Cut into 12 ¾-inch slices for the same Exchanges.
2. For a change, top with fresh peaches or berries, or serve it without any topping. It's delicious plain.
3. A special occasion recipe. Try it as a birthday cake with Cocoa Whipped Cream (see next recipe).

Sponge Cake with Cocoa Whipped Cream

Yield: 24 slices

Exchanges per slice:

    ½ Bread

    2 Fat

    2 Fruit

Estimated nutrients per serving:

CAL	193	FAT	9
CHO	25	Na	56
PRO	3	K	73

Ingredients

    1 PINT WHIPPING CREAM

    ⅓ CUP DUTCH PROCESS COCOA

    ⅔ CUP SIFTED CONFECTIONER'S SUGAR

    1 TEASPOON VANILLA

    1 10-INCH TUBE SPONGE CAKE

Method

1. Whip cream until it stands in peaks.
2. Combine cocoa and sugar. Beat into whipping cream. Add vanilla before last final strokes.
3. Cut sponge cake horizontally into 2 layers. Spread ¼ of topping on bottom layer. Replace top layer. Frost top and sides with remaining whipped cream. Refrigerate until served.

Applesauce Cupcakes

Yield: 12 cupcakes
Exchanges per cupcake:
    ½ Bread
    2 Fat
    1 Fruit

Estimated nutrients per serving:

CAL	174	FAT	10
CHO	18	Na	239
PRO	3	K	52

Ingredients

  ½ CUP MARGARINE
  1 EGG
  ¼ CUP SUGAR
 1½ CUPS SIFTED FLOUR
  1 TEASPOON BAKING SODA
  ¼ TEASPOON SALT
  1 TEASPOON CINNAMON
 1½ TEASPOONS NUTMEG
  1 CUP UNSWEETENED APPLESAUCE
  1 TEASPOON VANILLA
  ¼ CUP CHOPPED WALNUTS

Method

1. Preheat oven to 375° F.
2. Cream margarine until fluffy.
3. Beat eggs and sugar; add to margarine and blend.
4. Sift together dry ingredients. Add to margarine mixture alternately with applesauce, mixing well after each addition.
5. Stir in vanilla and nuts.
6. Spoon into 12 cupcake pans sprayed with vegetable pan spray.
7. Bake 15 to 20 minutes.

Sugarless Cookies

Yield: 32–34 cookies
Exchange per 2-cookie
serving:

    1 Bread
    1½ Fat

Estimated nutrients per serving:

CAL	144	FAT	8
CHO	15	Na	116
PRO	3	K	192

Ingredients

1¾ CUPS FLOUR
  2 TEASPOONS BAKING POWDER
 ½ TEASPOON SALT
 ½ TEASPOON CINNAMON
 ¾ CUP ORANGE JUICE
 ½ TEASPOON GRATED ORANGE RIND
 ½ CUP MINUS 1 TABLESPOON VEGETABLE OIL
  1 EGG
 ½ CUP CHOPPED WALNUTS
 ½ CUP RAISINS

Method

1. Preheat oven to 375° F.
2. Combine dry ingredients. Add remaining ingredients; mix well.
3. Drop by teaspoon on ungreased cookie sheet to make 32–34 cookies.
4. Bake about 15 to 20 minutes.
5. When done, remove from pan and cool.

Variations:

1. Add ¼ teaspoon ground cloves for a spice drop.
2. Instead of raisins, add ½ cup chopped or whole cranberries.

Sesame Cookies

Yield: 48 cookies
Exchanges per 2-cookie
serving:

    1 Bread
    1 Fat

Estimated nutrients per serving:

CAL	122	FAT	6
CHO	15	Na	110
PRO	2	K	12

Ingredients

  2 CUPS SIFTED FLOUR
  ¼ TEASPOON SALT
1½ TEASPOONS BAKING POWDER
  ⅔ CUP MARGARINE
  ⅔ CUP SUGAR
  2 EGGS
  1 TEASPOON VANILLA
  1 TABLESPOON SKIM MILK
  2 TABLESPOONS SESAME SEEDS

Method

1. Preheat oven to 375° F.
2. Sift together flour, salt, and baking powder.
3. Cream margarine and sugar. Add eggs, vanilla, and milk. Beat well.
4. Add dry ingredients; mix thoroughly.
5. Drop dough by teaspoons on ungreased baking sheet. Yield should be 48 cookies.
6. Flatten cookies with fork dipped in water. Sprinkle with sesame seed.
7. Bake 10 to 12 mnutes.

Oatmeal Cookies

Yield: 60 cookies

Exchanges per 2-cookie
serving:
    1 Bread
    1 Fat
    ½ Fruit

Estimated nutrients per serving:

CAL	134	FAT	6
CHO	18	Na	243
PRO	2	K	85

Ingredients

- ¾ CUP VEGETABLE SHORTENING
- ½ CUP BROWN SUGAR
- ½ CUP GRANULATED SUGAR
- 1 EGG
- ¼ CUP WATER
- 1 TEASPOON VANILLA
- 1 CUP FLOUR
- 1 TEASPOON SALT
- ½ TEASPOON BAKING SODA
- 1 CUP RAISINS
- 3 CUPS ROLLED OATS, QUICK COOKING OR REGULAR

Method

1. Preheat oven to 350° F.
2. Beat together shortening, sugars, egg, water, and vanilla until creamy.
3. Combine flour, salt, and soda. Add to creamed mixture. Add raisins and rolled oats. Mix well.
4. Drop by rounded teaspoonfuls onto ungreased cookie sheet; makes 5 dozen cookies.
5. Bake 12 to 15 minutes.

Peanut Butter Balls

Yield: 8 balls (4 servings)

Exchanges per 2-ball serving:
- ½ Medium-Fat Meat
- 1 Bread
- 1 Fat

Estimated nutrients per serving:

CAL	165	FAT	9
CHO	16	Na	148
PRO	5	K	222

Ingredients

- ¼ CUP PEANUT BUTTER
- ¼ CUP SKIM MILK, DIVIDED
- ¼ CUP RAISINS
- 4 GRAHAM CRACKERS (2-INCH SQUARE), BROKEN IN PIECES
- 1 TEASPOON VANILLA
  DASH CINNAMON

Method

1. Cream peanut butter with 2 tablespoons milk until well blended.
2. Add remaining ingredients. Mix well.
3. Drop on aluminum foil or wax paper in balls about 1 inch in diameter.
4. Place in freezer until ready to serve.

Bitter Chocolate Mounds

Yield: 30 pieces
Exchanges per 2-piece serving:
    ½ Bread
    ½ Fat
    ½ Fruit

Estimated nutrients per serving:

CAL	79	FAT	3
CHO	12	Na	49
PRO	1	K	92

Ingredients

    2 OUNCES BAKING CHOCOLATE
    1 OUNCE SEMISWEET CHOCOLATE BITS (ABOUT 65 PIECES)
  ½ CUP RAISINS
3½ CUPS RICE CEREAL

Method

1. Melt chocolate in heavy pan over low heat, stirring occasionally.
2. Add raisins and cereal; stir to coat.
3. Drop by tablespoons onto cookie sheet covered with waxed paper. Make 30 mounds. Chill in refrigerator.

Once chilled, these may be kept at room temperature.

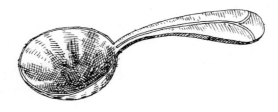

Plain Yogurt

Yield: 4 cups (4 servings)
Exchanges per 1-cup serving:
   1 Milk
   1 Fat

Estimated nutrients per serving:

CAL	161	FAT	5
CHO	17	Na	182
PRO	12	K	575

Ingredients

  1 QUART 2% LOW-FAT MILK
  ⅓ CUP NONFAT DRY MILK POWDER
  ¼ CUP PLAIN YOGURT WITH ACTIVE CULTURES (READ LABEL)

Method

1. Preheat oven to 275° F.
2. Mix low-fat and dry milk together. Heat to 180° F. Cool to 110° F.
3. Mix a little of the warm milk into yogurt; stir into bulk of warm milk. Pour into clean casserole dish. Cover.
4. Turn oven off. Put yogurt mixture in oven. Let sit, undisturbed, for 4 to 8 hours. The longer it sits, the tarter it will be.
5. Remove from oven. Divide into 1-cup (8-ounce) serving portions, using glass, plastic, or waxed paper containers with covers (or seal with foil, Saran, or waxed paper lids). Refrigerate.

Note: This yogurt can be used as starter in future preparations if used within five days. It can also be used for recipes in this book which require plain, low-fat yogurt.

Enriched Yogurt*

Yield: 7 cups (14 servings)
Exchanges per ½-cup serving:
   1 Milk

Estimated nutrients per serving:

CAL	93	FAT	1
CHO	14	Na	176
PRO	8	K	569

Ingredients

  1 ENVELOPE GELATIN
  1 CUP WATER, DIVIDED
  3 CUPS NONFAT DRY MILK
  3 CUPS WATER
  1 TALL CAN EVAPORATED SKIM MILK (13 OUNCES)
  1 CAN WATER (13 OUNCES)
 ¼ CUP SUGAR
  3 TABLESPOONS PLAIN YOGURT, WITH ACTIVE CULTURES

Method

1. Preheat oven to 275° F.
2. Sprinkle gelatin over ½ cup cold water in 2-quart casserole.
3. Bring remaining ½ cup water to boil. Add to gelatin. Stir to dissolve.
4. Add remaining ingredients. Mix well. Be sure all ingredients are lukewarm (about 110°). Excessive heat and cold can inactivate yogurt.
5. Cover casserole. Put in oven. Turn off oven.

6. Remove from oven after 4 to 8 hours. Longer incubation results in tarter taste. Stir well. Refrigerate in individual serving cups with lids.
7. 3 tablespoons of this yogurt can be used as starter in future preparation if used within five days.

Serving suggestion: Top with any fruit or vegetable. Be imaginative. Try pureed prunes, spiced pumpkin, applesauce, crushed pineapple.

*Note: This is a richer, more concentrated yogurt than the Plain Yogurt. For recipes calling for plain low-fat yogurt, *do not* use this recipe. See Plain Yogurt recipe.

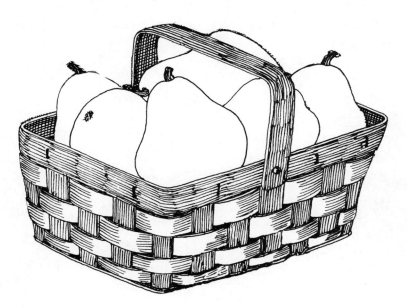

Beverages

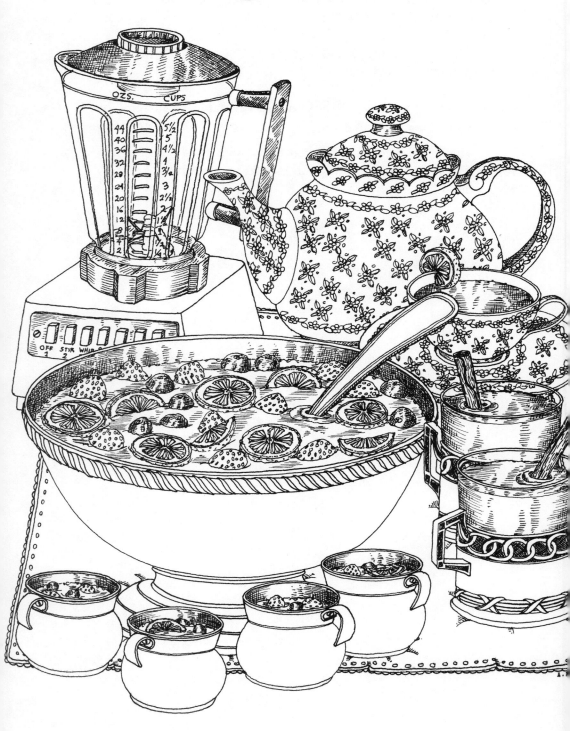

Do you yearn for something different to drink with a meal or as a snack? Some of these recipes yield one or two servings. Others, such as Hot Spiced Cider, Grape Sparkle, or the Strawberry-Grapefruit Punch, are suitable for serving a crowd.

Hot Spiced Tea

Yield: 4 cups (6 servings)
Exchanges per ⅔-cup serving:
    Free

Estimated nutrients per serving:

CAL	2	FAT	—
CHO	1	Na	2
PRO	—	K	6

Ingredients

    4 CUPS WATER
    1 CINNAMON STICK
    2 WHOLE CLOVES
    1 LONG STRIP LEMON PEEL (4 INCHES)
    1 LONG STRIP ORANGE PEEL (6 INCHES)
      DASH OF NUTMEG
3 or 4 TEA BAGS (OR AS DESIRED)

Method

1.   In saucepan combine all ingredients except tea.
2.   Simmer for 5 to 10 minutes.
3.   Add tea bags, or tea leaves if preferred. Let steep to taste.
4.   Serve hot, or chill for iced tea.

Apple Tea Cooler

Yield: ⅔ cup (1 serving)
Exchanges per ⅔-cup serving:
    1 Fruit

Estimated nutrients per serving:

CAL	40	FAT	—
CHO	10	Na	1
PRO	—	K	83

Ingredients

  ⅓ CUP APPLE JUICE, UNSWEETENED
  ⅓ CUP TEA
     ICE CUBES
     LEMON WEDGE (OPTIONAL)

Method

1. Mix apple juice and tea.
2. Serve over ice cubes. Garnish with lemon wedge if desired.

Hot Spiced Cider

Yield: 4 cups (8 servings)
Exchanges per ½-cup serving:
    1 Fruit

Estimated nutrients per serving:

CAL	44	FAT	—
CHO	11	Na	4
PRO	—	K	86

Ingredients

2⅔ CUPS APPLE CIDER
1⅓ CUPS WATER
  1 CINNAMON STICK
  ½ TEASPOON WHOLE CLOVES
  ½ TEASPOON WHOLE ALLSPICE
    ORANGE OR LEMON SLICE FOR GARNISH (OPTIONAL)

Method

1. Simmer ingredients (except fruit slices) together in saucepan for 10 minutes. Strain.
2. Serve hot with orange or lemon slice and a cinnamon stick garnish.

Grape Sparkle

Yield: 4 cups (8 servings)
Exchanges per ½-cup serving:
1 Fruit

Estimated nutrients per serving:

CAL	44	FAT	—
CHO	11	Na	1
PRO	—	K	79

Ingredients

2 CUPS UNSWEETENED GRAPE JUICE
2 TABLESPOONS LEMON JUICE
2 CUPS CLUB SODA

Method

1. Combine juices in quart pitcher.
2. Slowly pour club soda down side of pitcher. Stir gently to mix.
3. Serve over ice.

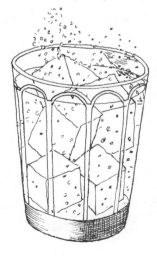

Grapefruit Fizz

Yield: 2 cups (2 servings)
Exchanges per 1-cup serving:
    1 Fruit

Estimated nutrients per serving:

CAL	50	Fat	—
CHO	12	Na	1
PRO	1	K	200

Ingredients

    1 CUP UNSWEETENED GRAPEFRUIT JUICE
    1 CUP CLUB SODA

Method

1. Pour juice into pitcher. Pour soda slowly down side of pitcher. Mix gently.
2. Pour over ice in chilled glasses.

Variations:

1. Substitute 1 cup orange juice for grapefruit juice.
   (Makes 2 1-cup servings = 1 Fruit Exchange)
2. Substitute 1 cup pineapple juice for grapefruit juice.
   (Makes 3 ⅔-cup servings = 1 Fruit Exchange)

Strawberry-Grapefruit Punch

Yield: 8 cups (8 servings)
Exchanges per 1-cup serving:
    1 Fruit

Estimated nutrients per serving:

CAL	42	Fat	—
CHO	10	Na	NA
PRO	1	K	NA

Ingredients

    1 10-OUNCE PACKAGE UNSWEETENED FROZEN
      STRAWBERRIES
    3 CUPS UNSWEETENED GRAPEFRUIT JUICE
    1 LITER (4½ CUPS) CLUB SODA

Method

1. Blend strawberries and juice in blender until smooth. Pour in pitcher or punch bowl.
2. Slowly pour club soda down side of pitcher. Stir gently to mix.

Variation: Use orange juice instead of grapefruit juice.

Tomato Appetizer

Yield: 3 cups (6 servings)
Exchanges per ½-cup serving:
    1 Vegetable

Estimated nutrients per serving:

CAL	28	FAT	—
CHO	6	Na	292
PRO	1	K	286

Ingredients

  3 CUPS TOMATO JUICE
  2 TABLESPOONS LEMON JUICE
½ TEASPOON SUGAR
¼ TEASPOON CELERY SALT
½ TEASPOON WORCESTERSHIRE SAUCE
  6 LEMON SLICES (OPTIONAL)

Method

1. Combine juice and seasonings.
2. Chill. Garnish with lemon slice.

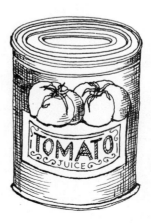

Tomato-Kraut Cocktail

Yield: 3 cups (6 servings)
Exchanges per ½-cup serving:
    1 Vegetable

Estimated nutrients per serving:

CAL	24	FAT	—
CHO	5	Na	531
PRO	1	K	213

Ingredients

    2 CUPS TOMATO JUICE
    1 CUP SAUERKRAUT JUICE

Method

1. Combine juices.
2. Pour over crushed ice.

Variation: For a change, serve hot.

Banana Shake

Yield: 2 cups (2 servings)
Exchanges per 1-cup serving:
    ½ Milk
    ½ Bread
    ½ Fat
    1 Fruit

Estimated nutrients per serving:

CAL	138	FAT	2
CHO	25	Na	91
PRO	5	K	506

Ingredients

    1 CUP SKIM MILK
    ½ CUP VANILLA ICE MILK
    1 SMALL RIPE BANANA

Method

1. Blend milk and ice milk in blender at high speed until smooth.
2. Add banana. Blend 2 or 3 seconds.
3. Serve immediately.

Strawberry Shake

Yield: 2¼ cups (3 servings)
Exchanges per ¾-cup serving:
    ½ Milk
    ½ Fruit

Estimated nutrients per serving:

CAL	81	FAT	1
CHO	14	Na	70
PRO	4	K	303

Ingredients

    1 CUP SKIM MILK
    ¾ CUP FRESH STRAWBERRIES (OR FROZEN
        UNSWEETENED, PARTIALLY THAWED)
    ½ CUP VANILLA ICE MILK

Method

1. Put milk and berries in blender container.
2. Blend 8 to 10 seconds.
3. Add ice milk. Blend until smooth.
4. Serve immediately.

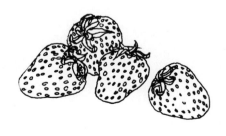

Orange-Yogurt Nog

Yield: 3 cups (4 servings)
Exchanges per ¾-cup serving:
    ½ Milk
    1 Fat
    1 Fruit

Estimated nutrients per serving:

CAL	120	FAT	4
CHO	15	Na	76
PRO	6	K	295

Ingredients

    1 CUP ORANGE JUICE
    1 8-OUNCE CARTON PLAIN, LOW-FAT YOGURT
    1 TABLESPOON HONEY
    2 EGGS
    4 ICE CUBES
      NUTMEG AS DESIRED

Method

1. Place all ingredients, except ice and nutmeg, in blender container.
2. Cover and blend at high speed until frothy.
3. Add ice cubes, one at a time, blending smooth after each addition.
4. Pour into 4 glasses. Add sprinkle of nutmeg. Serve immediately.

Strawberry Nog

Yield: 4 cups (4 servings)
Exchanges per 1-cup serving:
 ¾ Milk
 ½ Fat

Estimated nutrients per serving:

CAL	79	FAT	3
CHO	8	Na	60
PRO	5	K	217

Ingredients

 1 8-OUNCE CARTON PLAIN, LOW-FAT YOGURT
 ½ CUP SKIM MILK
 1 CUP FRESH OR UNSWEETENED FROZEN STRAWBERRIES
 1 EGG
 ¼ TEASPOON VANILLA
3 or 4 ICE CUBES

Method

1. Place all ingredients, except ice, in blender container.
2. Cover and blend at high speed until frothy.
3. Add ice cubes, one at a time, blending smooth after each addition.
4. Pour into 4 glasses. Serve immediately.

Variation: 1 cup fresh or unsweetened frozen peaches and ¼ teaspoon almond extract may be used in place of strawberries and vanilla.

Recipes Using Artificial Sweetner

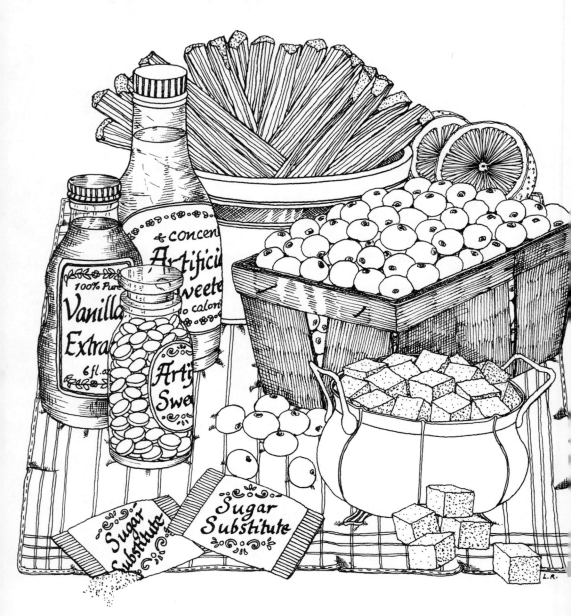

A few fruits are so tart that they must be sweetened. For these fruits, as well as rhubarb and cranberries, the recipes include artificial sweetener.

The many brands of artificial sweetener available do not all have the same sweetening power. The recipes, therefore, indicate the amount of sweetener in terms of its sweetness in comparison with sugar. Be sure to read the label to know how much to add.

Fresh Lemonade

Yield: 4 cups (4 servings)
Exchanges per 1-cup serving:
    Free

Estimated nutrients per serving:
CAL   12   FAT   —
CHO   3   Na   8
PRO   —   K   58

Ingredients

⅔ CUP FRESH LEMON JUICE
3⅓ CUPS WATER
    ARTIFICIAL SWEETENER EQUIVALENT TO ½ CUP SUGAR

Method

1. Mix all ingredients.
2. Chill and serve with ice.

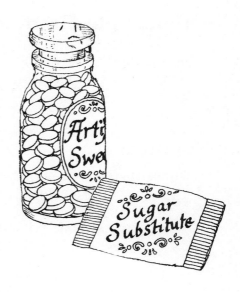

Orange-Lemon-ade

Yield: 4 cups (4 servings)
Exchanges per 1-cup serving:
    1½ Fruit

Estimated nutrients per serving:

CAL	64	FAT	—
CHO	15	Na	6
PRO	1	K	276

Ingredients

  ⅓ CUP FRESH LEMON JUICE
  2 CUPS FRESH OR RECONSTITUTED FROZEN ORANGE
     JUICE
1⅔ CUPS WATER
     ARTIFICIAL SWEETENER EQUIVALENT TO ⅓ CUP SUGAR

Method

1. Mix all ingredients.
2. Chill. Serve over ice.

Pineapple-Cranberry Relish

Yield: 2 cups (16 servings)
Exchanges per 2-tablespoon
serving:
    Free

Estimated nutrients per serving:

CAL	16	FAT	—
CHO	4	NA	13
PRO	—	K	31

Ingredients

  ½ POUND CRANBERRIES (2 CUPS)
  1 CUP CRUSHED PINEAPPLE, CANNED IN JUICE, WELL
     DRAINED
     LIQUID ARTIFICIAL SWEETENER EQUIVALENT TO
  ½ CUP SUGAR

Method

1. Wash cranberries, removing stems and soft berries.
2. Grind raw cranberries.
3. Add pineapple and sweetener.

Serving suggestion: This relish is tart, a good accompaniment to turkey or any other meat. It will keep well in the refrigerator for use with many meals.
Note: The recipe may be doubled to use the entire 1-pound package of cranberries. However, cranberries may be frozen in a plastic bag for later use. Consider freezing some for the months when they are not available.

Cranberry Punch

Yield: 2 quarts (16 servings)
Exchanges per ½-cup serving:
    1 Fruit

Estimated nutrients per serving:

CAL	36	FAT	1
CHO	8	Na	1
PRO	1	K	71

Ingredients

  1 POUND CRANBERRIES
     WATER AS NEEDED
  1 6-OUNCE CAN FROZEN ORANGE JUICE CONCENTRATE
     ARTIFICIAL SWEETENER EQUIVALENT TO 2
     TABLESPOONS SUGAR

Method

1. Wash cranberries, removing stems and soft berries. Cook according to package instructions until berries are soft.
2. Chop in blender or put through food mill. Add 2 cups water.
3. Strain through cheesecloth or several thicknesses of nylon net.
4. Add orange juice concentrate and artificial sweetener. Dilute with enough water to make 6 cups.

Rhubarb Sauce

Yield: 2 cups (4 servings)
Exchanges per ½-cup serving:
   Free

Estimated nutrients per serving:

CAL	8	FAT	—
CHO	2	Na	1
PRO	—	K	151

Ingredients

  2 CUPS RHUBARB, CUT INTO 1-INCH PIECES
  ½ CUP WATER
     ARTIFICIAL SWEETENER EQUIVALENT TO ¼ CUP SUGAR,
     OR TO TASTE

Method

1. Cook rhubarb with water about 10 minutes or until tender.
2. Remove from heat and add artificial sweetener.
3. Serve warm or chilled.

Rhubarb may be a finishing touch for a meal or a tangy breakfast fruit. One recipe tester froze some in a plastic container for her husband's lunch box.

Hot Cocoa

Yield: 2 cups (2 servings)
Exchanges per 1-cup serving:
   1 Milk

Estimated nutrients per serving:

CAL	105	FAT	1
CHO	15	Na	128*
PRO	9	K	487

Ingredients

1½ TABLESPOONS COCOA
  2 CUPS SKIM MILK
    DASH SALT*
    VANILLA TO TASTE (OPTIONAL)
    ARTIFICIAL SWEETENER EQUIVALENT TO 1
    TABLESPOON SUGAR

Method

1. Mix cocoa with ½ cup milk. Stir in remaining milk. Cook over low heat, stirring constantly until mixture comes to boil.
2. Remove from heat. Add salt, vanilla, and artificial sweetener.

*Na content of salt not included in estimate.

Vinegar Dressing

Yield: 1 cup (8 servings)
Exchanges per 2-tablespoon
serving:
    Free

Estimated nutrients per serving:

CAL	8	FAT	—
CHO	2	Na	68
PRO	—	K	34

Ingredients

  1 CUP WINE VINEGAR
    LIQUID ARTIFICIAL SWEETENER EQUIVALENT TO 1
    TABLESPOON SUGAR
 ½ TEASPOON SWEET BASIL
    DASH THYME
 ¼ TEASPOON SALT
    DASH FRESH GROUND PEPPER

Method

1. Mix all ingredients in pint jar.
2. Cover and store in refrigerator. Shake well before using.

Miscellaneous

Sauces can change the ordinary to the sublime. The ever-versatile white sauce—spiced and seasoned to taste—adds endless variety served on vegetables, over boiled new potatoes, or with leftover meats, canned tuna, or diced hard-cooked eggs as a main dish served on toast. The mushroom and cheese variations offer additional ways to serve a familiar food in a new way.

Tartar Sauce

Yield: 1 cup (16 servings)
Exchanges per 1-tablespoon serving:

    1½ Fat

Estimated nutrients per serving:

CAL	65	FAT	7
CHO	1	Na	53
PRO	1	K	15

Ingredients

  ½ CUP MAYONNAISE
  ½ CUP DAIRY SOUR CREAM
  1 TEASPOON GRATED ONION
  1 TABLESPOON MINCED DILL PICKLE
  1 TEASPOON MINCED FRESH PARSLEY

Method

1. Mix all ingredients.
2. Refrigerate.

White Sauce and Variations

Yield: 1 cup (8 servings)
Exchanges per 2-tablespoon
serving:
    1 Fat

Estimated nutrients per serving:

CAL	43	FAT	3
CHO	3	Na	119
PRO	1	K	54

Ingredients

  2 TABLESPOONS MARGARINE
  2 TABLESPOONS FLOUR
 ¼ TEASPOON SALT
 ⅛ TEASPOON PEPPER
  1 CUP SKIM MILK

Method

1. Melt margarine in saucepan over low heat.
2. Blend in flour, salt, and pepper.
3. Add milk, stirring constantly.
4. Remove from heat when sauce thickens and bubbles.

Variations:

For a thinner white sauce to serve over vegetables, increase milk to 2 cups or decrease margarine and flour to 1 tablespoon each. Two tablespoons of this thinner sauce may be considered as ½ Fat Exchange.

    For variations in texture and flavor, saute ¼ cup chopped onion or celery in margarine for white sauce, and then add flour. Each of these will increase the yield of 1 cup of sauce to 1⅛ cup. Adding ¼ cup of crisp sliced water chestnuts will increase 1 cup of sauce to 1¼ cups. Dry mustard (¼ teaspoon for 2 cups sauce) adds tang.

Serving suggestions: White sauce can be the basis of many do-it-yourself recipes. Combine it with almost any vegetable, meat, fish, or eggs for a tasty dish to serve on toast, rice, or pasta. Combine vegetable with a meat or meat substitute. Fold in pasta (spaghetti, macaroni, noodles) or rice or serve over toast, biscuits, corn bread, etc. The possibilities are endless.

Suggested amounts to combine with 1 cup of the basic White Sauce recipe:

VEGETABLES	Yield
1 10-ounce package frozen peas	2 cups
1 10-ounce package frozen chopped broccoli	2 cups
1 10-ounce package frozen chopped spinach	2 cups

MEAT AND OTHER PROTEIN-RICH FOODS	
4 hard-cooked eggs	1½ cups
1 2½-ounce jar sliced dried beef	1½ cups
2 cups diced ham	2 cups
1 7-ounce can tuna, drained	1¾ cups

For your Exchange calculations, 1 cup of the basic sauce is approximately equal to 1 Milk, 1 Bread, and 4 Fat Exchanges. Add Exchanges for the meat or vegetable you use in the recipe. Then divide the total Exchanges by the number of servings.

Cheese Sauce

Yield: 1½ cups (12 servings)   Estimated nutrients per serving:

Exchanges per 2-tablespoon serving

½ Vegetable

1 Fat

CAL	65	FAT	5
CHO	2	Na	138
PRO	3	K	39

Ingredients

    1 CUP WHITE SAUCE (SEE RECIPE)

    1 CUP GRATED CHEDDAR CHEESE (ABOUT 4 OUNCES)

    ¼ TEASPOON DRY MUSTARD

Method

1. To hot white sauce, add cheese and mustard.
2. Stir until melted.

Quick Cheese Sauce

Yield: 1¼ cups (10 servings)   Estimated nutrients per serving:

Exchanges per 2-tablespoon serving:

½ High-Fat Meat

½ Fat

CAL	87	FAT	7
CHO	1	Na	NA
PRO	5	K	NA

Ingredients

    2 CUPS DICED SHARP PROCESSED CHEESE (ABOUT 8 OUNCES)

    ⅓ CUP SKIM MILK

Method

1. Melt cheese in double boiler.
2. Slowly stir in milk.

Mushroom Sauce

Yield: 1½ cups (12 servings)
Exchanges per 2-tablespoon
serving:

    ½ Fat

Estimated nutrients per serving:

CAL	30	FAT	2
CHO	2	Na	79
PRO	1	K	36

Ingredients

- 2 TABLESPOONS MARGARINE
- 1 4-OUNCE CAN SLICED MUSHROOMS, DRAINED
- 1 TEASPOON GRATED ONION
- 2 TABLESPOONS FLOUR
- ¼ TEASPOON SALT
- ⅛ TEASPOON PEPPER
- 1 CUP SKIM MILK

Method

1. Melt margarine in small skillet. Add mushrooms and onion; saute until onions are tender.
2. Blend in flour, salt, and pepper.
3. Add milk, stirring constantly. Cook until mixture bubbles and thickens.

Serving suggestion: Serve over meat, vegetables, omelets, or toast.

Sauerkraut Relish

Yield: 2 cups (6 servings)
Exchanges per ⅓-cup serving:
    1 Vegetable

Estimated nutrients per serving:

CAL	16	FAT	—
CHO	4	Na	205
PRO	1	K	84

Ingredients

  1 CUP SAUERKRAUT, UNDRAINED
½ CUP CHOPPED ONION
¼ CUP CHOPPED GREEN PEPPER
½ CUP CHOPPED CELERY
  2 TEASPOONS VINEGAR
  2 TABLESPOONS WATER
  1 TABLESPOON SUGAR

Method

1. Mix vegetables.
2. Combine vinegar, water, and sugar; pour over other ingredients.
3. Refrigerate overnight. Stir occasionally.
4. Store, covered, in refrigerator. Relish will keep for 2 weeks in refrigerator.

Serving suggestion: Adds tang to roast beef or roast pork.

Suggested Menus
For Special Occasions

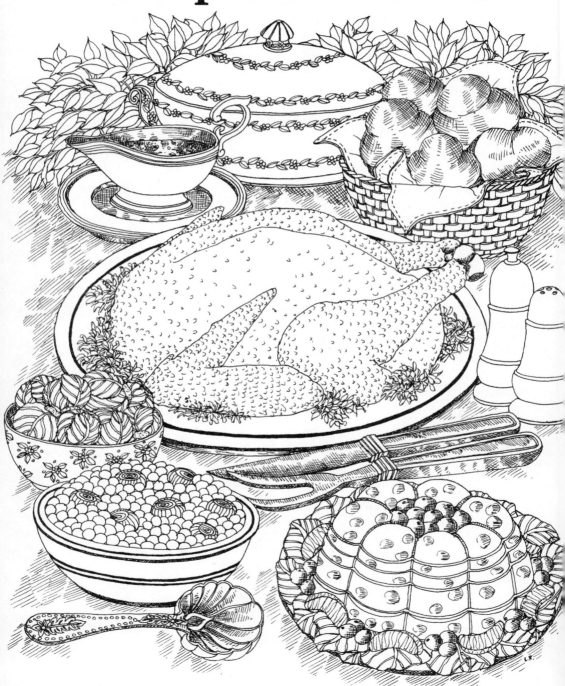

An appetizing menu, whether for the family or for a special occasion, is a combination of foods you enjoy. It provides eye appeal as well as a blend of flavors and textures. When someone in the family has a diabetic meal pattern, your menu planning may actually become easier because you have guidelines to encourage you to choose foods of several types.

These menus merely offer suggestions. Your own family preferences, your schedule, the seasonal availability of produce, and your own way with food, will inspire variations. The success of a dinner may depend less on its cost than on the table setting, choice of foods, and relaxed atmosphere.

The menus do not indicate portions because they were not written for an individual meal plan. The amounts and number of items to select will depend on the meal plan in your home.

The starred items may be found in the index.

SUMMER LUNCHEON

Fruited Chicken Salad*
Celery Hearts, Radishes, and Black Olives
Baking Powder Biscuits*
Apricot Sherbet*

FAMILY DINNERS

Macaroni and Cheese Custard*
Broiled Tomatoes*
Molded Green Salad*
Blueberry Pudding*

Grilled Halibut with Tartar Sauce*
Herb-stuffed Potato*
Green Beans with Slivered Almonds
Sliced Cucumber Salad
Cherry-Berry Compote*

Hearty Split Pea Soup*
French Bread
Cottage Cheese with Tomato Wedges
Peach Slices with Soft Custard Sauce*

CHICKEN EVERY SUNDAY

Gazpacho*
Sesame Chicken Breasts*
Whipped Potato
Orange Glazed Carrots*
Mixed Green Salad
Pineapple Snow*

TEEN PARTY

Hot Spiced Cider*
Cereal Party Mix*
Assemble-Your-Own Tacos*
Dill Pix Sticks
Strawberry Ice Milk Cones

BUFFET SUPPER

Lasagne*
Greek Salad*
Hard Rolls
Fresh Fruit Cup

AN INTERNATIONAL FLAIR

Chicken Egg Drop Soup*
Chinese Ginger Chicken* with Rice
Snow Peas
Head Lettuce with Vinegar
Minted Fresh Pineapple

AFTER THE GAME

Chili Con Carne*
Double Corn Muffins*
Tossed Salad
Baked Apple*

PATIO COOKOUT

Grilled Steak
Confetti Potato Salad*
Corn on the Cob
Cherry Tomatoes and Green Onions
Melon Balls

THE CHRISTMAS TABLE

Consomme
Roast Turkey
Bread Dressing*
Peas and Pearl Onions
Pineapple-Cranberry Relish*
Celery Hearts
Ambrosia*

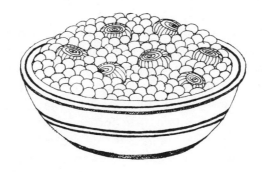

7 □ CALCULATING EXCHANGES FROM FOOD LABELS AND RECIPES

You've mastered the art of planning via the exchange system. Now you're ready to try your wings and to challenge your friendly neighborhood supermarket with its dazzling array of 8,000 food items, give or take a few hundred.

Can you cope? Can you match up your newly mastered art with the nutrition information provided on package labels in the store.

This skill is not for the faint of heart, but it pays dividends. By learning the language of food labels, you can add incredible variety to your meals. At the store, you will be better equipped to decide whether or not foods like frozen pizza or broccoli in cheese sauce are nutritionally wise. And at home you will be able to figure out whether or not the recommended portion is right for your meal plan.

Is a food overloaded with sugar or salt? Is the carbohydrate or fat content way out of line compared to the amount of protein provided? A quick look at nutrition information will tell you the answers. If, for example, a food has 30 grams of carbohydrate and only 2 grams of protein, you can quickly see that the food is overloaded with carbohydrate and may not provide adequate nutrients. Now, look at the ingredients. Do one or more forms of sugar make up too large a portion of the product? That's the case with many cakes and fruit-flavored yogurts, for example.

What about Exchanges? Is that can of stew a good choice for lunch. You can use nutrition labels to find out how one serving translates into diabetic Exchanges. Calculating Exchanges requires

318

some time at home with pencil and paper or a calculator. The more calculating you do, however, the easier it will become.

Before you begin calculating by yourself, scan "The Wise Calculator," which explains some of the logic behind calculations for packaged foods.

THE WISE CALCULATOR

1. As important as knowing *how* to calculate Exchanges is understanding the reasoning behind the process. Before you start calculating Exchanges for a lot of foods, discuss a few examples with a diet counselor, and ask questions. If you don't know any dietitians or nutritionists, contact your local American Diabetes Association Affiliate for help in locating one.

2. The first step in calculating Exchanges for packaged foods is listing the main ingredients and deciding which Exchange Lists they correspond to. You can tell which ingredients are the main ones by their order on the label: the first ingredient listed is the most predominant (by weight), the second ingredient is the next most important, and so on. The first three or four ingredients probably contribute most of the carbohydrate, protein, fat, and calories; but also consider the other foods on the list. If a lot of the items fall into one category (such as sugars), they might compose more of the product than they seem to at first.

3. If the product you're working with is mostly composed of complex carbohydrate (bread, cereal, pasta, flour, or certain vegetables), you will generally start your calculations by determining the number of Bread Exchanges, followed by the next most prominent Exchange Group. Foods whose carbohydrate comes mainly from "sugars" are often exchanged as Fruits. If the product is mostly protein, you'll start with Meat Exchanges, and if it's mostly made of milk, you'll start with Milk Exchanges.

4. As a rule of thumb, when you figure out how many Exchanges there are in 1 serving, you may round off fractions; although, of course, fractions are more accurate. If the fraction is less than ½, drop it. If it's more than ½, round up to the nearest whole

number. However, if the fraction is equal or close to ½, count it as ½.

5. To check your calculations, look at how many Exchanges you have determined are in 1 serving of the packaged food and, using the table, add up the number of grams of carbohydrate, protein, and fat, and the calories, in those Exchanges. Your total should vary very little from the numbers on the nutrition label. If you vary by approximately 2–3 grams each of carbohydrate, protein, or fat *per meal,* or 15–20 calories, you need to do no further calculating. Per day, you will not want to vary from your meal plan by more than 5 grams in any category, and by more than 40 calories.

6. If you eat many convenience foods and work them into your meal plan, the "leftover" amounts of carbohydrate, protein, fat, and calories can add up. Therefore, avoid using too many prepared foods in the same day or even the same week. Sticking as closely as possible to your meal plan is important.

HOW TO CALCULATE EXCHANGES
Before you follow the steps below, carefully read the following table of values which lists the carbohydrate, protein, fat, and Calorie content of the six lists in "Exchange Lists for Meal Planning" (see Chapter 3). Keep the chart handy; you'll want to refer to it later.

SUMMARY OF NUTRIENT AND CALORIC COMPOSITION OF EXCHANGE LISTS

Exchange List	CARB(g)	PRO(g)	FAT(g)	CAL
Milk (non-fat)	12	8	–	80
Vegetables	5	2	–	25
Fruit	10	–	–	40
Bread (including cereals and starch vegetables)	15	2	–	70
Lean Meat	–	7	3	55
Medium-Fat Meat	–	7	5	75
High-Fat Meat	–	7	8	100
Fat	–	–	5	45

Now look at the specific steps. We'll use a macaroni and cheese dinner as an example.

The nutrition label for the macaroni and cheese dinner reads:

Serving Size   ¾ cup
Calories   240
Protein (grams)   10
Carbohydrate (grams)   32
Fat (grams)   7

And the main ingredients listed are:

Macaroni
Cheddar Cheese

METHOD 1

Step 1. List the main ingredients and determine which Exchange groups they fall into.

MAIN INGREDIENTS	EXCHANGE GROUPS
Macaroni	Bread
Cheddar Cheese	High-Fat Meat

SERVING	CARB(g)	PRO(g)	FAT(g)	CAL
¾ cup	32	10	7	240

Step 2. From the package, list the grams of carbohydrate, protein, and fat in 1 *suggested serving*. List the calories too.

Step 3. Figure out, and then list, the number of Exchanges in the most prominent Exchange group—in this case, Bread. (Macaroni is in the Bread Exchange because carbohydrate is the main ingredient. Bread Exchanges have the highest carbohydrate content.)

To find the number of Bread Exchanges, divide the number of grams of carbohydrate in 1 *serving* by the number of carbohydrate grams in 1 *Exchange* (15 grams) taken from the *Summary of Nutrient and Caloric Composition of Exchange Lists table*. *(32 g. ÷ 15 g. = 2.13 Bread*, which rounds off to 2 Bread Exchanges.) Since 1 Bread Exchange has 15 grams of carbohydrate, 2 grams of protein, no fat, and 70 calories (see *Values* table), then 2 Bread Exchanges have 30 grams of carbohydrate (2 × 15 g.), 4 grams of protein (2 × 2 g.), and 140 calories (2 × 70).

Step 4. Subtract the amounts of carbohydrate, protein, fat, and calories you get in Step 3 from the amounts listed on the label to see how much of each would be "left over" if you were to count 1 portion of macaroni and cheese as just 2 Bread Exchanges. Too many grams and calories are "left over" (see *The Wise Calculator*, page 319).

	CARB(g)	PRO(g)	FAT(g)	CAL
Amount on label	32	10	7	240
Less 2 breads	30	4		140
(Results of subtracting)	2	6	7	100

Go to the next major Exchange group on your list and repeat steps 3 and 4 until you have almost no carbohydrate, protein, fat, and calories left over.

Step 5. The next food group here is High-Fat Meat, which is a protein Exchange food. To see how many Exchanges you have, divide the *remaining protein* (6 grams) by the amount of protein in *1 Exchange* (7 grams.) (6 g. ÷ 7 g. = .0857 Meats, which rounds off to 1 High-Fat Meat Exchange.) From the nutrient summary table, you know that 1 High-Fat Meat has 7 grams of protein, 8 grams of fat, and 100 calories.

	CARB(g)	PRO(g)	FAT(g)	CAL
1 High-Fat Meat	–	7	8	100
(Results of subtracting) from results in Step 4)	2	−1	−1	–

The totals vary little from the numbers on the nutrition label. You need do no further calculation.

Step 6. List Exchanges for 1 serving.

¾ cup = 2 Bread Exchanges and 1 High-Fat Meat Exchange

Different diet counselors use different approaches to calculating Exchanges. The following approach avoids using fractions. Work with a diet counselor to determine the approach that's easier for you.

METHOD 2

Step 1. List the main ingredients and determine which Exchange Groups they fall into.

MAIN INGREDIENTS	EXCHANGE GROUP
Macaroni	Bread
Cheddar Cheese	High-Fat Meat

SERVING	CARB(g)	PRO(g)	FAT	CAL
¾ cup	32	10	7	240

Step 2. From the package, list the grams of carbohydrate, protein, and fat in 1 serving. List the calories, too.

Step 3. List the amounts of carbohydrate, protein, fat, and calories in 1 *Exchange* of the main food group, in this case, Bread.

SERVING	CARB(g)	PRO(g)	FAT(g)	CAL
1 Bread	15	2	–	70

Step 4. List the amounts of carbohydrate, protein, fat, and calories in 1 *Exchange* of the second main food group, in this case, High-Fat Meat.

SERVING	CARB(g)	PRO(g)	FAT(g)	CAL
1 High-Fat Meat	–	7	8	100

Step 5. Add up the values for Steps 3 and 4 to see if all of the carbohydrate, protein, fat, and calories are close to the number on the label.

SERVING (Results of adding)	CARB(g)	PRO(g)	FAT(g)	CAL
	15	9	8	170

Step 6. If, as in this case, the totals are not close to the original label (see Step 2), you have to do more calculating. Subtract the numbers in Step 5 from the numbers on the label (Step 2). (This shows you how much is "left over.")

SERVING	CARB(g)	PRO(g)	FAT(g)	CAL
(Results of subtracting)	17	1	−1	70

Step 7. Now determine which Exchange Group the remaining amounts of carbohydrate, protein, fat, and calories most closely approximate. In this case, approximately 1 Bread Exchange remains.

SERVING	CARB(g)	PRO(g)	FAT(g)	CAL
1 Bread	15	2	–	70

Step 8. Subtract the amounts in Step 7 from the amounts in Step 6 to see if you need to do more calculating. Here, you can see that the "leftover" grams of carbohydrate, protein, and fat are negligible.

SERVING	CARB(g)	PRO(g)	FAT(g)	CAL
(Results of subtracting)	2	1	−1	–

Step 9. List Exchanges for 1 serving.

¾ cup = 2 Bread Exchanges and 1 High-Fat Meat Exchange.

A WORD ABOUT PORTION SIZES

If you expect to eat more servings than just one, multiply all amounts by the number of servings you plan to have. For instance, if you planned to eat two servings of macaroni and cheese, you would multiply all numbers by 2.

1 suggested serving (¾ cup) = 2 Bread Exchanges and 1 High-Fat Meat Exchange

2 servings (6/4 cup, or 1½ cups) = 4 Bread Exchanges and 2 High-Fat Meat Exchanges

If you planned to eat half of a serving, you would divide the numbers of Exchanges by 2. (If you wanted to eat a third of a portion, you would divide by 3; if you wanted a quarter of a portion, you would divide by 4, and so on.)

1 suggested serving (¾ cup) = 2 Bread Exchanges and 1 High-Fat Meat Exchange

½ serving (⅜ cup) = 1 Bread Exchange and ½ High-Fat Meat Exchange

If you wanted to change your serving size to equal 1 Bread Exchange of macaroni and cheese, you would divide everything by the number of Exchanges in 1 suggested serving to find out how large your new portion would be. Since you now have 2 Bread Exchanges in one suggested serving, and you want to eat only 1 Exchange's worth, divide all values by 2.

1 suggested serving (¾ cup) = 2 Bread Exchanges and 1 High-Fat Meat Exchange

1 new portion = (¾ cup ÷ 2 = ⅜ cup) = 1 Bread Exchange and ½ High-Fat Meat Exchange

Here are a few more examples.

CORNBREAD MIX

1. INGREDIENTS	EXCHANGE GROUPS
Flour	Bread
Cornmeal	
Margarine	Fat

	SERVING	CARB(g)	PRO(g)	FAT(g)	CAL
2. One serving:	1 square	18	2	6	135
3. $18 \div 15 = 1\ 1/5$, rounded off to 1 Bread	1 Bread	15	2	–	70
4. (Results of subtracting)		3	–	6	65
5. $6 \div 5 = 1\ 1/5$, rounded off to 1	1 Fat	–	–	5	45
6. (Results of subtracting)		3	–	1	25

7. One serving (1 square) = 1 Bread and 1 Fat Exchange

ITALIAN STYLE VEGETABLES

1. INGREDIENTS	EXCHANGE GROUPS
Green Beans⎫ Red Pepper ⎬ Onion ⎭	Vegetable
Chick Peas ⎫ Corn Starch ⎭	Bread
Olives	Fat

	SERVING	CARB(g)	PRO(g)	FAT(g)	CAL
2. One serving:	3.3 ounces	9	2	1	45
3. $9 \div 15 = 3/5$, rounded off to ½ Bread	½ Bread*	7.5	1	–	35
4. (Results of subtracting)		1.5	1	1	10

One serving (3.3 ounces) = ½ Bread

---

*Bread is used because many people will have more Bread Exchanges in their meal plan. This can also be calculated in terms of vegetables. 2 Vegetables = 10 grams of carbohydrate, 4 grams of protein, no fat, and 50 calories.

MINIATURE RAVIOLI IN MEAT SAUCE

1. INGREDIENTS	EXCHANGE GROUPS
Flour	Bread
Cracker Meal	Bread
Tomatoes	Vegetable
Beef	Medium-Fat Meat
Cheddar Cheese	High-Fat Meat

	SERVING	CARB(g)	PRO(g)	FAT(g)	CAL
2. One serving	7½ ounces	32	9	6	220
3. 32 ÷ 15 = 2 2/15, rounded off to 2 Breads	2 Breads	30	4	–	140
4. (Results of subtracting)		2	5	6	80
5. 5 ÷ 7 = 5/7, rounded off to 1	1 Medium-Fat Meat	–	7	5	75
6. (Results of subtracting)		2	−2	1	5

7. One serving (7½ ounces) = 2 Breads and 1 Medium-Fat Meat

Learning how to use nutrition labels for improved nutrition and variety can make diabetes management easier. With just a bit of effort, you can become a smarter consumer and can add flexibility to your daily meal planning.

7. Since you are familiar with the basic process of exchanging foods, you will see that some foods can be broken down into a variety of Exchanges to fit individual meal plans and that deciding which Exchanges to use is often a matter of judgment. Different "calculators" may come up with different Exchanges for the same food and each be "right." For example, consider miniature ravioli in meat sauce, a product discussed earlier in the chapter. We concluded that 1 serving had 2 Bread Exchanges and 1 Medium-Fat Meat Exchange. However, by the manufacturer's calculations the ravioli dish has 2 Bread Exchanges, 1 Vegetable Exchange, and

1 Lean-Meat Exchange. Comparing values, you can see that both are close.

	CARB(g)	PRO(g)	FAT(g)	CAL
1 serving (7½ ounces) =	32	9	6	220
(a) 2 Breads + 1 Medium-Fat Meat =	30	11	5	215
(b) 2 Breads + 1 Vegetable + 1 Lean Meat =	35	13	3	220

The first way is more exact with respect to carbohydrate, protein, and fat content; but the second way is more exact with respect to calories (energy). Energy is an important consideration also, and either Exchange calculation can be used in your meal plan.

8. Some high-carbohydrate foods (such as mixed vegetables) that you might expect to treat as Vegetable Exchanges, can be calculated in terms of Bread Exchanges to fit into your meal plan. (Notice that "Exchange Lists for Meal Planning" lists mixed vegetables on the Bread List.) This is acceptable because, like foods on the Vegetable Exchange List, foods on the Bread List provide 2 grams of protein and other nutrients. Look, for example, at Tomato Bisque, which you might expect to treat as a vegetable.

	CARB(g)	PRO(g)	FAT(g)	CAL
1 serving (11 ounces) made with water:	29	2	4	160
Counting 1 serving as 2 Breads + ½ Fat:	30	4	2.5	163
(Results of subtracting)	−1	−2	1.5	−3

9. A less obvious possibility, though an acceptable practice, is to calculate desserts in terms of Bread Exchanges. Since the first ingredient on the package is often sugar, you would be correct in assuming that the food most closely fits into the "Fruit Exchange"

category. Bread Exchanges are used sometimes, however, because very few people have more than 1 Fruit Exchange allotted for any given meal, and most desserts would count as more than 1 Fruit Exchange. Obviously, calculating in this way allows you to accommodate an occasional dessert for special times. Keep in mind, however, that nutritionally (in terms of protein and vitamins) these foods are not really equivalent to true Bread Exchanges and should be substituted into your meal plan only once in a while.

10. When in doubt, ask questions.

SUPERMARKET STRATEGY

1. Copy the basic Exchange List of Values table onto ruled paper or an index card and keep it in your wallet for easy reference while you shop.

2. Once you have calculated Exchange values for a specific food, keep a chart that lists the food name, serving size, Exchange values, and Calories. To avoid losing the list, keep one copy with your Exchange List table and keep a duplicate at home, perhaps taped to the inside of a cabinet door.

3. Remember that foods produced by different manufacturers may have different ingredients in different proportions, so the Exchange and Calorie values for one food (such as macaroni and cheese) may vary from brand to brand; also, manufacturers sometimes change the makeup of their products. Check the ingredients and nutrition information regularly.

4. At the store, inspect the ingredients list to see if any of the ingredients are inappropriate or present in too large quantities. Look particularly at:

(a) *The first few ingredients.* Remember that the most prominent ingredients are listed first. However, different forms of the same type of foods, such as sugar, can be listed separately and may comprise quite a bit of the product.

(b) *Sugar, by any of its names.* If you just look for the word "sugar" on the ingredients list, you may be misled. Aside from table sugar (sucrose), other forms of sugar include glucose, dextrose, maltose, fructose, corn syrup, corn sweetener, molasses, brown sugar, date sugar, "raw" sugar, invert sugar, lactose, and honey. The ending "ose" is a clue that the food is a sugar. Also be on the lookout for sugary ingredients, such as raisins and dates. If there is only one of these sugars, low down on the list, the amount may be minor, but a number of them can add up to a lot of sugar. If some form of sugar is listed in the first three ingredients and the carbohydrate content of the food is high, add that food to your diet only after checking with your physician.

Foods containing fructose, sorbitol, and mannitol, which are also sweeteners, should be used only if the calories are calculated into the diabetic meal plan and if their use has been discussed with a health professional. The foods containing this form of sugar are not "free" foods because the form of sugar used has almost equal calorie content to table sugar.

(c) *Salt, an often hidden ingredient.* People who have been told to watch their salt intake can use the ingredient statement for clues about the salt content. Much of the salt we eat comes from food additives used as preservatives and flavorings. When the label includes salt, monosodium glutamate, sodium citrate, sodium hydroxide, sodium propionate, and sodium nitrate, use the product sparingly or avoid it altogether. Canned vegetables, cured meats (bacon, sausage, cold cuts), pickles, sauerkraut, and frozen convenience dinners have high sodium levels, as do many salted snack foods and nuts. These foods need to be limited if sodium intake is restricted.

(d) *Fat, in its better and worse forms.* If you want to avoid saturated fats, avoided animal fats (such as butter), foods that contain coconut oil or palm oil, and unspecified types of vegetable oil (chances are it's saturated). Liquid vegetable oils have less saturated fat than partially hydrogenated or hardened oils, so look for margarine containing liquid oils. Cholesterol, which comes from animal fats, is harder to judge. Most labels that list cholesterol list it to point out that the levels are low.

5. Look at the vitamins listed on the nutrition label. When nutrition information is supplied, the lower part of the label lists the

percentage of U.S. Recommended Daily Allowances of selected important vitamins and minerals. The recommended U.S. RDA's for people aged four and older are:

Vitamin	U.S. RDA
Vitamin A	5,000 International Units
Vitamin C (ascorbic acid)	60 milligrams
Thiamine (Vitamin B_1)	1.5 milligrams
Riboflavin (Vitamin B_2)	1.7 milligrams
Niacin	20 milligrams
Calcium	1.0 grams
Iron	18 milligrams

6. Know your metrics. Sometimes nutrients are listed in metric units, not ounces. You should know that:

1 pound = 454 grams (g)
1 ounce = 30 grams (g)
1 gram = 1000 milligrams (mg)

7. Avoid foods with no nutrition labels. Unless the manufacturer sends you nutrition information (upon request, many will), you have no way of calculating Exchange Values or determining carbohydrate, protein, fat, or calorie content. Fortunately, although not all packaged foods are required by law to include nutrition information, about 75 percent of them do. Foods that claim to have special dietary properties, such as being low in calories or low in fat, must carry nutrition labels.

In summary, there can be several different ways to calculate the Exchange values for any one food product. For instance, carbohydrate is found in the Milk and Fruit Exchange groups as well as the Bread and Vegetable Exchange groups. To be most correct, read the ingredients list and put each ingredient into its Exchange group. Use this information to determine which Exchange groups are best to use for your calculation.

Remember that other brands and other foods may have different serving sizes, different ingredients, and/or different nutritional values. Check the label *carefully* of each individual food product.

It is helpful to keep a record of your Exchange values for the various food products. However, food manufacturers do change their "recipes." Periodically check your copy of the ingredients and the nutrition information label with the one currently on the package.

Practice makes the figuring of exchange values for convenience foods easier. If you need more help or information, ask your diet counselor. Then, enjoy the time saved by using a macaroni and cheese mix or a frozen pizza!

NEW FOODS

Many new formulated foods (such as powdered creamer) that imitate or replace traditional foods are appearing on the market. Nutrition labeling can help you learn what nutrients these foods contain and how they can be used.

Read the label or write to the manufacturer for information about the carbohydrate, protein, and fat content per serving of these products. Or, for more specific information, contact a registered dietition in private practice or in a hospital or nutrition clinic.

SPECIAL DIET FOODS

Modified foods are prepared for use in many different kinds of special diets; low-cholesterol egg products are an example. Some are lower in calories than comparable regular foods, others may be lower in sodium. Nutrition labels can be used to compare the calories and nutrients in special diet foods with those in regular foods to determine which ones are acceptable for use on your particular diet.

DIETETIC FOODS

What about dietetic foods? Many foods are labeled "dietetic," but not all of them are for the diabetic. "Dietetic" means "pertaining to diet." "Diabetic" means "pertaining to diabetes." The words may sound alike, but they do not mean the same thing.

There are various kinds of dietetic foods. Some of them are:

1. Those in which sugar has been left out or in which a substitute has replaced it.
2. Those in which salt has been left out.
3. Those using a different kind or amount of fat than usually used.
4. Those which leave out an ingredient to which an allergy may exist.

Therefore, a food described as "dietetic" does not necessarily have fewer calories. Some do and some do not. You need to read the label carefully.

Let calories be your guide for choosing how much of these dietetic foods to use. It is generally recommended that you add not more than 30 to 40 extra calories to your day's meal plan *from any food,* including dietetic foods. For example:

1 tablespoon low-calorie jelly	3 calories
2 sticks "sugar-free" chewing gum (5 calories per stick)	10 calories
2 teaspoons powdered nondairy creamer (8 calories per teaspoon)	16 calories
	29 calories

Two or three extra calories in a serving may not seem like much, but they do add up. Eventually, those extra calories could exceed the total calories in the day's meal plan.

Ask your diet counselor for advice about using dietetic foods in the meal plan. If you question a product, it is better not to use it. Instead, use dietetic foods only occasionally and enjoy the foods of the Exchange Lists every day.

CALCULATING EXCHANGES FROM RECIPES

Your treasured family recipes needn't be put on the shelf because of diabetes or carbohydrate control. Instead, many can be calculated into Exchanges. It's easy as 1–2–3–4:

1. List all ingredients used in the recipe and the amounts.

2. Identify the Exchange group for each item and the number of Exchanges. (A list of common household equivalents is given in the Appendix.) For example, 1 ounce *cooked* meat = 1 Exchange.

3. Figure the total for each Exchange group.

4. Divide the total number of Exchanges in each group by the total number of servings for the recipe to find the number of Exchanges for one serving. Round to the nearest ½ Exchange. (Amounts less than ½ need not be counted; amounts over ½ round up to the next whole number.)

The following examples show how this procedure works.

Southern Oven Hash yields: 4 ½-cup servings

INGREDIENTS	EXCHANGES						
	Milk	Veg.	Fruit	Bread	Meat	Fat	Free
Ground beef, *cooked*, 1 cup					4		
Potatoes, *cooked*, 1 cup				2			
Onion, ground, ¼ cup							X
Parsley, ¼ cup							X
Worcestershire sauce, 2 teaspoons							X
Evaporated milk, ½ cup	1					2	
Bread crumbs, ¼ cup				1			
Butter, melted, 1 tablespoon						3	
TOTAL EXCHANGES	1			3	4	5	
TOTAL EXCHANGES FOR ONE SERVING	¼			¾	1	1¼	

Exchanges per serving: 1 Bread   1 Meat   1 Fat

In accordance with the rule stated in Step 4, the Milk Exchange of ¼ per serving is less than ½ so is dropped; the ¾ bread is more than ½ so is rounded to the next whole number, which is 1; 1 Meat remains 1 Meat; and 1¼ Fat becomes 1 Fat.

When a meat is cooked it loses approximately ¼ of its raw weight. When a recipe calls for raw meat, subtract 25 percent before determining the number of Exchanges. For example:

1 pound ground meat = 16 ounces

$$\underline{-4 \text{ ounces}} \text{ (¼ raw weight)}$$
12 ounces

When regular sugar is used in baking, calculate it as a Fruit Exchange. One tablespoon of granulated sugar contains about 10 grams of carbohydrate. For example, a recipe for Granny's Cocoa Oat Refrigerator Morsels would look like this when calculated:

Granny's Cocoa Oat Refrigerator Morsels yield: 72 Cookies

INGREDIENTS	EXCHANGES						
	Milk	Veg	Fruit	Bread	Meat	Fat	Free
Flour, 1½ cups (2½ tablespoons = 1 Bread)				10			
Baking soda, 1 teaspoon							X
Salt, 1 teaspoon							X
Shortening, 1 cup (16 tablespoons = 1 cup, 3 teaspoons = 1 tablespoon)						48	
Brown sugar, 1 cup (1 tablespoon = 13 grams CHO)			20				
Granulated sugar, 1 cup (1 tablespoon = 11 grams CHO)			18				

INGREDIENTS	EXCHANGES						
	Milk	Veg	Fruit	Bread	Meat	Fat	Free
Eggs, 2					2		
Oatmeal, 3 cups (1 cup = 4 Bread)				12			
Pecans, ½ cup						8	
Coconut, 1½ cups						12	
TOTAL EXCHANGES (72 cookies)			38	22	2	68	
TOTAL EXCHANGES FOR 1 SERVING (1 cookie)			½	⅓	0	1	
If you eat 2 cookies, you must mutiply by 2:			1	⅔	0	2	

Exchanges per 2 cookies:
1 Fruit* 1 Bread* 2 Fat

*Each cookie contains 1⅓ teaspoons sugar. The carbohydrate in this recipe, although called Fruit Exchange, is derived from sugars. These carbohydrate sources do not contain the vitamins normally associated with Fruit Exchanges.

SUMMARY

The methods described in this chapter should help you adapt your family's favorite convenience food and recipes to Exchanges. The Appendix provides tools for you to do more of this on your own. The Supplemental Exchange List includes a variety of foods not on the Exchange Lists for Meal Planning, and The Guide for Common Measurements should help you in your recipe calculations.

If you get stumped, call your diet counselor!

8 □ DINING OUT

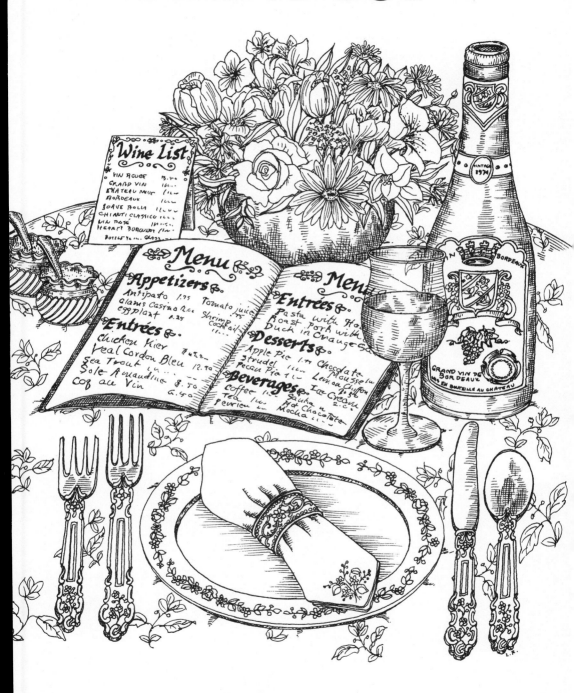

Anyone with diabetes can eat out by following simple guidelines.*
1. Be familiar with the meal plan. If you aren't, carry a copy with you.
2. Familiarize yourself with the foods and portion on each Exchange List.
3. Become familiar with serving sizes by practicing at home. Faithful measuring will teach you to recognize portions.
4. If portion sizes are too large, ask for a doggie bag and save the leftovers for the next day.
5. Don't hesitate to ask questions about how a food is prepared. If something you want is not on the menu, ask for it.
6. If you are insulin-dependent, you must eat on schedule. If you think there will be a wait for a table or the service will be slow, the family member with diabetes may want to eat part of his or her usual meal before going to the restaurant.
7. Although what and how much you eat depends on your meal plan, foods that are generally suitable and those to avoid are listed on the following pages.

FOODS TO ORDER

Appetizers	Tomato juice, unsweetened fruit juice. Clear broth, bouillon, consomme. Celery, radishes, dill pickles, etc. Fresh fruit, unsweetened.
Meat, Poultry, Fish	Roasted, baked, or broiled meat, poultry, fish, or seafood. Broiled foods may be available on request, but expect a 20-minute wait for them. For an extra treat, remember to look for regional specialties, such as seafood on the coasts. Ask that gravy be omitted and trim excess fat from meats. If a food should arrive unexpectedly breaded, peel off the outer coating. If the serving exceeds the meal plan portion, ask for a doggie bag.

*The material in this chapter is adapted from *Diabetes Forecast,* May–June 1978.

FOODS TO ORDER (continued)

Eggs	Poached, boiled, scrambled.
Potatoes and Substitutes	Mashed, baked, boiled, steamed potatoes. Rice, noodles.
Fats	Butter, margarine, salad dressing, bacon, cream, sour cream. (Remember also to count the fat used on vegetables in the kitchen. Count it as 1 Fat Exchange.)
Salads	Tossed vegetable, head lettuce, sliced tomatoes. Request that the dressing be served separately or choose a lemon wedge or vinegar. Cottage cheese is part of the meat allowance.
Breads	Plain whole wheat or enriched bread or toast. Rolls, biscuits (watch the size!). Crackers. Bread Dressing (⅓ cup = 1 Bread and 1 Fat Exchange). Other substitutes for 1 Bread Exchange: 2 9-inch-long bread sticks; 4 melba toast rectangles or 8 rounds; 3 Rye Krisp; ½ bagel; ½ hot dog bun (1 if small—about 1 ounce); ½ hamburger bun (most full-size buns = 2 Exchanges); 1 6-inch tortilla or taco shell; ½ English muffin.
Vegetables	Stewed, steamed, boiled. (If vegetables are not listed on the menu, ask if any are available.)
Desserts	Fortunately, desserts are usually priced separately. You might ask for: Fresh fruit or fruit juice. Ice cream, occasionally (½ cup scoop = 1 Bread and 2 Fat Exchanges). Or, plan to have an apple for eating in the car on the way home.
Beverages	Coffee, tea. Milk, according to the meal plan. Diet soft drink if available.

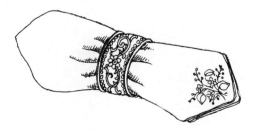

FOODS TO AVOID

Appetizers	Cream soups, thick soups. Sweetened juices. Canned fruit cocktail. Seafood cocktail (unless less meat is eaten later).
Meat, Poultry, Fish	Fatty, fried, and breaded foods. Meats in cream sauce, barbecued meat. Stews and casserole-type dishes (these are better eaten at home so you know what is in them).
Eggs	Fried, creamed.
Potatoes and substitutes	Fried, french-fried, creamed, escalloped, au gratin.
Fats	Gravy, fried foods, creamed foods.
Salads	Coleslaw and other salads with dressings. These are fine at home, but may have too much dressing in a restaurant. Canned fruit or gelatin salads.
Breads	Sweet rolls, coffee cake.
Vegetables	Creams, escalloped, au gratin.
Desserts	Puddings, custard, pastry. Sweetened fruits.
Beverages	Chocolate milk, cocoa, milk shakes, regular soft drinks

9 □ FAST FOODS

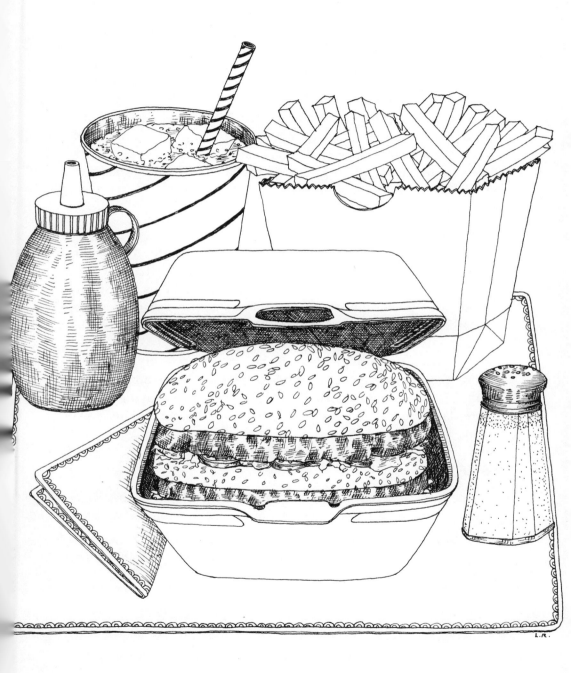

As you drive down Main Street, U.S.A., you see an extraordinary number of fast-food restaurants eager for your business. Americans are a people on the go, and grabbing meals outside the home is now a part of our lifestyle.

But what do you do if you or someone in your family has diabetes? What if you're away from home, it's time to eat, and your only choices are fast-food restaurants? Or, what if your family just *likes* fast foods? These questions needn't pose a problem. As a general rule, people who have diabetes can eat where everyone else eats. They merely have to do some intelligent choosing. Here are some guidelines and an Exchange List for fast foods to make that choosing easier.*

KNOW THE DIET

Insulin-dependent diabetics should try to choose foods that most closely approximate their allotted Exchanges, or whatever foods their diet allows. They should avoid high-sugar items unless these foods are specifically eaten just before intense exercise. and remember that calorie needs are different at meal times than at snack times.

Noninsulin-dependent diabetics who are trying to lose weight should pay special attention to calorie values and avoid high-sugar, high-fat, high-calorie foods. This may mean saying no to an extra-large burger and yes to a regular-sized burger and juice, skim milk, or tea.

SIZE UP PORTIONS

Contents of food may not be standardized in restaurants that are not part of a chain. In independent sandwich and submarine shops, for

*The material in this chapter is adapted from *Diabetes Forecast,* July–August 1979.

example, the amount of fillings and dressings, as well as the size and weight of breads, can vary. Nutrition values and Exchanges for the average tuna, roast beef, and cold-cut submarine sandwich are listed on the chart at the end of this chapter. But remember that a particular sandwich may vary considerably from the norm. Also, consider that a tuna sub may have 700 calories. Even if the sandwich is an average size, splitting it with a friend can be a good idea.

SKIP THE SWEETS

Avoid obviously sweet foods such as shakes and pies, and choose foods that more or less fit into the personal food pattern.

BE CHOOSY

Even if inappropriate foods are part of a package offering, a diabetic person can choose *not* to eat them. If, for example, the coleslaw is dripping with mayonnaise, skip it.

IF IN DOUBT, "GUESSTIMATE"

If you come across an unfamiliar food or a food not listed on the chart, try to break it down into the ingredients that it's composed of and figure out the number of Bread, Meat, and Fat Exchanges. Is there any mayonnaise, oil, or salad dressing—and how much? Is there meat, fish, or cheese—and how much? Don't underestimate! If a food is fried, you'll have to add an estimate of 2 to 3 Fat Exchanges. Is there a vegetable or fruit? Even if the meal has no hot vegetable, it may come with coleslaw or lettuce and tomato on the side.

Many people ask about the Exchanges for sandwiches made on pita, or Syrian pocket bread. The bread on such sandwiches may vary from 1½ to 2 ounces (or approximately 1⅓ to 2¼ Bread

Exchanges, and 100 to 160 calories). After you determine the Bread Exchange, the process for estimating exchanges is the same as for any other sandwich. Ask yourself "What's inside?" and "How much?"

PRACTICE MEASURING

If you're really unsure of how large the portions are, find a quiet time at home to get our your food scale, cups, and spoons and train your eye to judge.

INCLUDE VARIETY

Remember that to provide all daily nutritional needs, salad, vegetables, fruit, milk, and whole-grain items should be included. Such foods will add a variety of vitamins, minerals, and fiber to the diet of any age group. Many fast foods tend to be high in saturated fat, cholesterol, and salt.

FAST-FOOD EXCHANGE

The figures on the following Exchange List should help you to make intelligent choices. Some of the values listed are based on actual laboratory analysis; others have been approximated on the basis of similar foods because exact figures are not available. Although we continue to learn more about the nutritional values of fast foods, our information about many of these foods is still incomplete.

If your favorite food isn't here, try to compare it to a similar food. A roast beef sandwich, for example, would be similar to a hamburger. Also, many unlisted foods can be calculated by using your regular Exchange List. Just be sure to gauge portions accurately.

	NUTRITIONAL VALUES				EXCHANGES		
	CARB(g)	PRO(g)	FAT(g)	CAL	BREAD	MEAT (med.)	FAT *
ARTHUR TREACHER'S (Fish, chips, coleslaw)							
3-piece dinner	91	38	65	1100	6	4	9
2-piece dinner	83	28	51	905	5½	2½	8
BURGER CHEF							
Hamburger	23	12	12	250	1½	1	1½
Cheeseburger	24	14	17	304	1½	1½	2
Double hamburger	28	20	15	325	2	2½	½
Double cheeseburger	24	24	26	434	1½	3	2
Big Shef	41	25	30	535	2¾	3	3
Super Shef	39	29	37	600	2½	3½	4
Skipper's Treat	39	29	37	604	2½	3	4½
Rancher Platter	44	30	38	640	3	3½	4
Mariner Platter	85	32	24	680	5½	3	2
French Fries	25	3	9	187	1½	–	2
Milk shake, chocolate	48	9	9	310	3	½	1
BURGER KING							
Hamburger	29	15	13	290	2	1½	1
Hamburger with cheese	30	18	17	350	2	2	1
Double meat hamburger	30	25	22	420	2	3	1
Double meat hamburger with cheese	32	30	31	530	2	4	2
Whopper	50	26	36	630	3½	3	4
Double Beef Whopper	52	44	52	850	3½	5	5
Whopper with cheese	52	32	45	740	3½	3½	5
Double Beef Whopper with cheese	54	50	60	950	3½	6	5
Whopper Jr.	31	15	20	370	2	1½	2

*If Fat Exchanges seem too low, check meat calculations; fat content may be included there.

	NUTRITIONAL VALUES				EXCHANGES		
	CARB(g)	PRO(g)	FAT(g)	CAL	BREAD	MEAT (med.)	FAT*
BURGER KING (continued)							
Whopper Jr. with cheese	32	18	25	420	2	2	3
Whopper Jr. with double meat	33	25	29	490	2	3	3
Whopper Jr. double meat pattie with cheese	34	28	34	550	2	3	2½
Whaler	44	23	31	550	3	2	4
Whaler with cheese	45	28	40	650	3	3	4½
Steak sandwich	58	35	19	540	4	4	—
Onion rings	29	3	16	270	2	—	3
French fries	25	3	11	210	1½	—	2
Milk shake, chocolate	57	8	10	340	4	—	2
Milk shake, vanilla	52	8	11	340	3½	—	2

NOTE: New sandwiches have been added. Burger King may have figures.

	CARB(g)	PRO(g)	FAT(g)	CAL	BREAD	MEAT (med.)	FAT*
KENTUCKY FRIED CHICKEN (Fried chicken, mashed potato, coleslaw, rolls)							
3-piece dinner Original	61	50	43	830	4	6	2½
3-piece dinner Crispy	74	54	62	1070	5	6½	6
2-piece dinner Original	51	35	28	595	3½	4	1½
2-piece dinner Crispy	40	37	40	665	2½	4½	3½
LONG JOHN SILVER (Fish, chips, coleslaw)							
3-piece dinner	100	55	63	1190	7	6	7
2-piece dinner	89	38	50	955	6	3½	6
McDONALD's							
Hamburger	31	14	9	260	1½	1	1½
Cheeseburger	31	16	13	306	2	2	1
Quarter Pounder	33	26	21	418	2	3	1
Quarter Pounder with cheese	34	31	29	518	2½	3½	2

Big Mac	44	21	32	550	3	2	4
Filet-O-Fish	34	15	23	402	2½	1½	3
French fries	26	3	11	211	2	–	2
Egg McMuffin	26	18	20	352	2	2	2
Pork sausage	trace	9	17	184	–	1	2½
Scrambled eggs	2	12	12	162	–	1½	1
Shake, chocolate	60	11	9	364	4	½	1
PIZZA HUT (Cheese pizza)							
Individual thick crust	143	71	19	1030	9½	6	–
Individual, thin crust	128	61	28	1005	8½	6	–
½ of 13-inch thick crust	113	65	21	900	7½	6	–
½ of 13-inch thin crust	103	50	26	850	7	5	–
1 slice (⅛ of pie)	26	12½	6½	225	2	2	–
½ of 15-inch thick crust	148	83	31	1200	10	7	–
½ of 15-inch thin crust	144	66	35	1150	9½	7	–
SUBMARINE, HERO GRINDER (8-inch sandwich)							
Italian cold cuts	60	36	26	620	4	4	1
Roast beef	55	46	22	600	3½	5	–
Tuna	55	41	34	700	3½	5	2
TACO BELL							
Bean Burrito	48	11	12	343	3	1	2
Beef Burrito	37	30	21	466	2½	3½	½
Beefy Tostada	21	19	15	291	1½	2½	½
Bellbeefer	23	15	7	221	1½	2	–
Bellbeefer with cheese	23	19	12	278	1½	2	½
Burrito Supreme	43	21	22	457	3	2	2½
Combination Burrito	43	21	16	404	3	2	1
Enchirito	42	25	21	454	3	3	1½
Pintos 'n Cheese	21	11	5	168	1½	1	–
Taco	14	15	8	186	1	2	–
Tostada	25	9	6	179	2	1	–

* If Fat Exchanges seem too low, check meat calculation; fat content may be included there.

10 □ BROWN BAG LUNCH

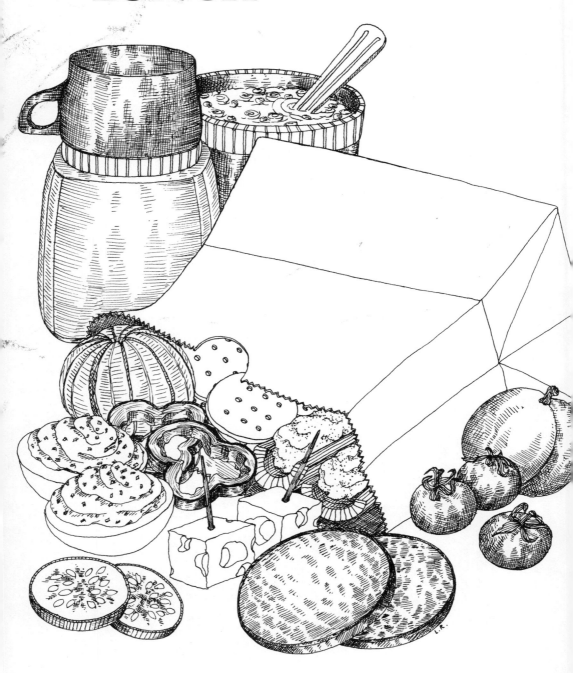

Portable meals are handy to take to school, to work, on picnics. A meal plan can be adapted to eating at home, in a restaurant, or anywhere. The brown bag lunch is especially flexible: there is no anxiety about slow service, no need to wait in lines, and no need to leave a tip.

There's more to lunch than a sandwich. Consider packing some of these in small plastic bags:

Cheese—a chunk or slices or cubes.

Peanut butter, stuffed into an apple or celery sticks.

Cottage cheese or cheese spread, in celery sticks or cucumber boats.

Tuna salad or egg salad, in celery sticks or cucumber boats, or wrapped in a lettuce leaf.

Chicken or turkey—cold cubes, wings, or drumsticks.

Meat, in pieces, slices, or cubes.

Meat loaf slices.

Hard-cooked eggs, plain or deviled.

Yogurt, plain or flavored with fresh fruit.

Ham slices rolled around cheese strips.

A plastic container can hold:

A chef's salad (carry salad dressing separately).

Cottage cheese with fresh fruit salad.

Shrimp salad in a tomato on lettuce.

How about using a wide-mouth vacuum bottle for:

Stew.

Baked beans.

Hearty Split Pea Soup.

Gazpacho.

Potato soup.

Spaghetti and meat.

Macaroni and cheese.

For sandwiches, vary the breads (check Bread Exchanges for size servings):

White, rye, whole wheat, French, Italian, or one of the

combination grain breads; English muffins, pita, rolls, corn bread, muffins, or biscuits; melba toast, crackers.

Also try different combinations such as the ones below. Keep in mind that mayonnaise, salad dressing, margarine, and butter are Fat Exchanges and may need to be measured.

Tofu with sliced cucumber and sesame seeds.

Tuna, chopped celery, and chopped apple moistened with a little mayonnaise.

Thin slices of roast beef, chicken, or ham with mustard or mayonnaise.

Luncheon meat, American cheese, thinly sliced dill pickle, and mustard on a hard roll.

Chicken, almonds, and bean sprouts combined with mayonnaise.

Mashed garbanzo spread with thinly sliced green pepper strips.

Corned beef, Swiss cheese, and thin slices of dill pickle on rye.

Peanut butter and chopped raisins or diced crisp bacon spread on whole wheat.

Hard-cooked egg, finely chopped then mixed with pimiento, celery, and green pepper moistened with mayonnaise.

Fish salad (made from previously broiled fish), mayonnaise, dill weed, and pepper.

Note: Be careful about holding highly perishable sandwich fillings at room temperature for long periods.

Plan the brown bag meal to include contrasts in flavors and textures. A meal is more appetizing when it contains something moist to offset dry food, tart foods to offset the sweet, and crisp foods as well as soft. Mayonnaise has been mentioned as one way to add moisture, but also consider mustard, lemon juice, and vinegar. Tomato and V-8 juices must be considered tart. Both vegetable and unsweetened fruit juices are sold in 6-ounce cans. Remember to make the appropriate exchange.

Beverages also add moisture. Coffee or tea can be carried hot or iced. Milk can be used if it is included in the meal plan.

Raw vegetables and pickles add crispness to the brown bag meal. Try carrot and celery sticks, radishes, green pepper strips, cut-up cauliflower, sliced cucumber, sliced onion, crisp lettuce, watercress, or cherry tomatoes.

Fresh fruits are easy to pack. As a change from the often-used apples, oranges, and bananas, try plums, apricots, or melon (pack in a plastic container), or pears when in season. Chilled canned fruits or a baked apple, pear, or peach travel well in a wide-mouth thermos. Remember to pack a plastic spoon too.

These additional suggestions will help make a brown bag meal easier to prepare and tastier to eat:

Meat sliced thin and then "stacked," are easier to bite than one thick slice on a sandwich.

Spread mayonnaise, margarine, or butter to the edge of the slice of bread so the moist filling won't make the bread soggy.

Wrap tomato slices, lettuce leaves, and other vegetables separately in clear plastic wrap or foil, so they stay crisp. Put them on the sandwich just before eating.

Score an orange and wrap in clear plastic wrap to make peeling easier.

Prepare raw vegetables the day or night before; wrap in foil or clear plastic wrap; refrigerate overnight. They are ready to add to the brown bag on a moment's notice.

Cut sandwiches in quarters; they are easier to eat and it seems like one is eating more.

Make a week's supply of sandwiches at one time. Meat, chicken, and peanut butter freeze well. Wrap individually; label with contents and date. Remove wrapped sandwich from the feezer in the morning. It will be ready to eat at lunch.

Whatever the occasion, a brown bag lunch does not need to be a slice of bologna between two slices of dry bread. Live it up! Use the variety in the Exchange Lists to the fullest extent. Make the lunches you pack a meal others will envy.

11 □ALCOHOL
AND DIABETES

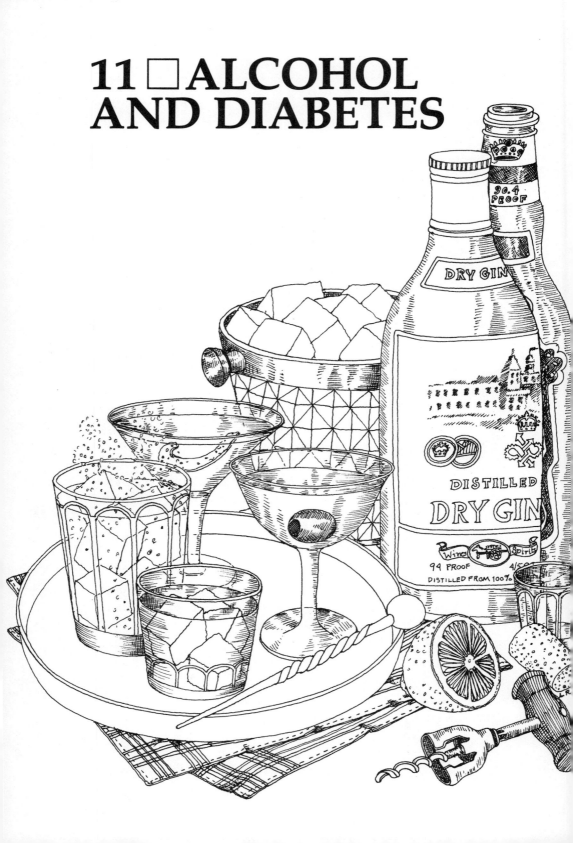

On occasion having a cocktail or a glass of wine is appropriate. Before using alcohol in a diabetic meal plan, speak with your physician and diet counselor. *When* and *how much* should be spelled out.

Alcohol is a source of many calories (7 calories per gram), but is essentially devoid of other nutrients. Beer and wine contain carbohydrate in addition to alcohol.

In the diabetic meal plan the amount of alcohol in the beverage is commonly figured in terms of Fat Exchanges, and the carbohydrate content of the beverage as Bread Exchanges. (See chart below for Exchange equivalents for alcoholic beverages.)

When alcohol is used in cooking, the alcohol evaporates while the food heats. Therefore the alcohol calories do not need to be counted. Usually the quantity of alcohol used is so small that the carbohydrate calories do not need to be counted either.

EXCHANGE EQUIVALENTS FOR ALCOHOLIC BEVERAGES

Amount	Type	Exchanges
1½ ounces	Liquor: gin, rum, whiskey, vodka, scotch (80 proof)	3 Fat Exchanges
12 ounces	Beer	1 Bread Exchange 2 Fat Exchanges
3 ounces	Dry wine (12% alcohol)	1½ Fat Exchanges
3 ounces	Sherry	½ Bread Exchange 2 Fat Exchanges

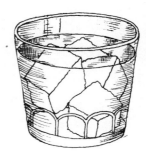

12 □ CANNING AND FREEZING FRUITS

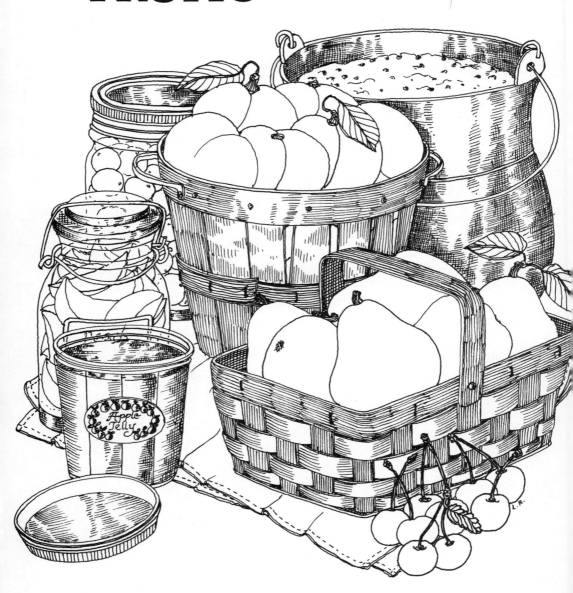

With summer comes the luxury of using fresh fruit. But the joy of having a variety of luscious fruits doesn't have to fade when the season ends. By canning or freezing fruits when in season—without sugar—you'll add variety to your diet all year long and stretch your food budget too.

The time to prepare fruit for storage is soon after harvesting. If you wait too long, the fruit begins to change color and lose flavor, and eventually it spoils.

CANNING

Canning involves heating fruits in sealed jars. If it's done in an organized way, it can be fun to do. The heating destroys bacteria, molds, and enzymes that promote spoilage, and the airtight sealing prevents foods from being recontaminated. Foods canned without sugar differ somewhat from those with sugar. Sugar helps to hold the shape, texture, appearance, and flavor of the original food. However, sugar is not *needed* to prevent spoiling.

The equipment needed is minimal. You'll need a water bath canner with a wide rack inside and a lid; jars, lids, and screwbands *made especially for home canning*; a saucepan, tongs, and several layers of thick cloth.

A boiling water bath canner rather than a steam-pressure canner may used with most fruits because fruits tend to be high in acid. These acids inhibit or prevent the growth of many of the microorganisms which cause spoilage and disease. The most common spoilage organisms associated with acid foods are yeasts and molds. They are easily destroyed at 212° F, the temperature of a boiling water bath. The same equipment is also used for highly acidic vegetables, such as tomatoes and pickles. The open-kettle method of canning is safe only for jams and jellies.

Before starting, check all equipment. Do *not* reuse lids with built-in sealing compound because they will not make airtight seals. Make sure all jars and screwbands have no nicks, cracks, chips, or rust; they must be in perfect condition.

To sterilize, put the jars and lids through the regular cycle of the dishwasher, or simply wash the jars in hot, soapy water. Rinse thoroughly. Wash and rinse all the lids and screwbands. Metal lids with sealing compound may need to be boiled or held in boiling water. Follow manufacturer's instructions. Then use tongs to remove.

For best quality in the finished product, select only fresh, firm, fully ripe, but not overripe, fruit.

Clean the fruit thoroughly. Peel, cut, and core or pit all fruits requiring it.

To prevent apples, apricots, peaches, and pears from discoloring, put the cut-up pieces in ascorbic acid or citric acid dissolved in water. (Buy these acids at your local grocery or drugstore; follow package directions.) If you prefer, instead of the acid you can use a solution of two tablespoons of vinegar or lemon juice mixed with two tablespoons of salt in one gallon of water. (This is not recommended as anti-darkening treatment for fruits to be eaten by the diabetic who also needs to limit sodium.) This method may alter the taste, but any change can be minimized by thoroughly rinsing the fruit before packing it into the jars.

Most fruits, except for berries, should be preheated before canning. When berries are preheated, the juice drains out. Although berries can be canned, freezing is a better method for preserving them.

When you're ready to can, drain the fruit and allow it to heat in a small amount of water. Heat peaches, pears, and apricots thoroughly; heat applesauce to simmering; heat berries (covered), cherries (covered), and plums to boiling; and boil apples for five minutes. Pack the hot fruit into clean, hot jars. Add enough boiling water or boiling unsweetened fruit juice to cover the fruit, leaving a half-inch of unfilled space in the jar. (The juice doesn't have to be made from the same kind of fruit you're canning. For example, peaches and pears may be packed in unsweetened grapefruit, apple, or pineapple juice. When available, white grape juice can also be used.) Leaving space in the jar ensures that the lid will seal. If jars are filled to the top, liquid may boil out during processing. Food particles may get trapped between the jar rim and the lid, causing a seal failure. If there is too much head space, however, some air may remain in the jar after processing, causing food at the top of the jar to darken, causing off-flavors and lowering vitamin retention, particularly in food at the top of the jar.

To remove air bubbles, insert a clean table knife gently between the side of the jar and fruit. Add more liquid to cover the fruit, if needed, remembering always to leave the half-inch head space. Repeat procedure until all of the fruit is used.

Wipe the top and threads of each jar with a clean, damp cloth. Place the hot lids on each jar, making sure that the sealing compound is next to the glass. If you're using a cap with a rubber ring, fit it in place around the neck of the jar. Place the hot lids on each jar and screw them on tightly by hand.

Note: *If the manufacturer's instructions for jars and lids differ from those given here, follow the directions of the manufacturer.*

Having the canning kettle filled with hot but not boiling water, place the sealed jars one at a time on a rack in the kettle. When all the jars are in place, add enough hot water so there are one or two inches above the jar tops; don't pour boiling water directly on glass jars. When the water begins to boil, reduce the heat to ensure a steady, gentle boil. This point, not when the jars are first put in, marks the beginning of the counting process. Process for the amount of time specified on the chart given below. The canner should be covered during the processing period. During the processing time check the water level periodically. If it begins to evaporate, add additional boiling water to maintain the water level above the jar tops.

When the jars have heated for the proper time, quickly remove them from the canner. Place them right-side up on several thicknesses of cloth a few inches apart and out of drafts.

Allow the jars to cool for 12 to 24 hours. Check each jar to make sure it's properly sealed. Lids are sealed if they are concave and will not move when pressed.

PROCESSING TIME (in minutes)

	pint	quart		pint	quart
Apples	15	20	Cherries	10	15
Berries	10	15	Peaches	20	25
Applesauce	10	10	Pears	20	25
Apricots	20	25	Plums	20	25

If the jar did not seal, the food has to be reprocessed. If you'd rather not reprocess, you may refrigerate the fruit and eat it within the next few days, just as you would any recently opened canned fruit.

Before you store jars away, remove the screwbands and save them for the next batch of canning. Label the jars, indicating the type of fruit, kind of liquid used, and the date. Sun and heat can spoil the fruit, even with the lids on, so store the jars in a cool, dark place. For best flavor and texture, use them within a year of processing.

Using non-nutritive sweeteners in canning is not recommended because they tend to take on a bitter taste when heated. If you want to use them, add just before serving.

If the fruit is to be used by only one or two members of the family, canning in pint-sized jars may help to prevent leftovers.

When fruit is packed in juice, remember to count the fruit juice as an additional Exchange.

FREEZING

Although fruits have better texture if packed in sugar or syrup, they may be frozen without sweetening. Blueberries, gooseberries, currants, cranberries, rhubarb, and figs freeze especially well without sugar.

Freezing keeps the fresh flavor and nutritive value of fruits better than other methods of preservation. Freezer temperatures— 0° F or below—retard the growth of bacteria, molds, and yeasts and slow down enzyme activity. But, unlike canning, freezing does not destroy microorganisms and enzymes.

To freeze berries, wash them quickly in cold water and drain well. Pack them, without added liquid, into heavy plastic freezer bags or plastic freezer boxes. Seal and freeze. Or spread a single layer of washed, well-drained berries on a cookie sheet or tray and put in freezer. When berries are frozen, transfer them to containers. Seal and return to freezer. The berries will be loose, so you can easily pour out as many or as few as you need.

Other fruits that are frozen without added liquid include grapes, rhubarb, melon balls, and pineapple wedges. Just pack them into containers, seal, and freeze.

To prevent peaches from darkening, pack them in water containing ascorbic acid. First, wash, pit, and peel the peaches. Pack peach halves or slices into plastic freezer boxes. Cover with cold water containing one teaspoon of crystalline ascorbic acid to each quart of water. (If you use a commercial anti-darkening preparation, follow the manufacturer's directions.) Press fruit down into the water with a small piece of crumpled parchment paper. Seal and freeze.

Leave frozen fruit in the sealed container to thaw. Thaw in the refrigerator or in a pan of cool water. Serve as soon as thawed. A few ice crystals in the fruit improve the texture for eating raw. For best quality, use frozen fruits within 8 to 12 months.

FOR MORE INFORMATION

For more information on canning and freezing, contact the Cooperative Extension Service office in your county. Your county Extension home economist can provide you with up-to-date bulletins on home food preservation and answer any specific questions you may have. You will find the Extension office number listed in the telephone directory along with other county office numbers.

13 □ SICK DAYS

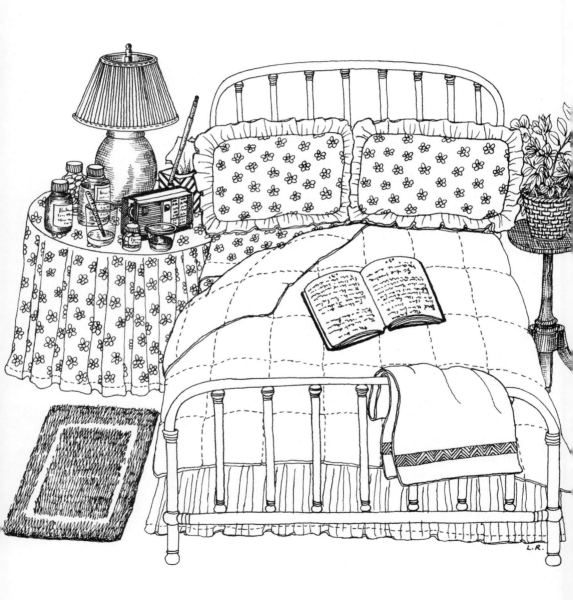

Everyone gets colds, the flu, and viruses—including people who have diabetes. However, for the diabetic, any illness has special implications.*

For example: The stress of illness, whether due to infection or to any other cause, can raise blood sugar and cause diabetes to go out of control; illness may cause loss of appetite or an insulin-dependent diabetic may incorrectly think that insulin is not required.

SICK DAY "DOs" FOR THE DIABETIC

1. Continue to take at least your usual dose of insulin and to test your urine.
2. If test results are high for sugar, test urine for ketones; report the presence of ketones to the doctor immediately.
3. If you use insulin, have a vial of regular insulin on reserve to use, if directed.
4. Eating and drinking are extremely important. If you have difficulty eating, switch to soft or liquid, easy-to-digest foods. (See suggestions on the following pages.) Attempt to follow your meal plan as closely as possible.
5. Report vomiting episodes to your doctor immediately.
6. Call your doctor if you're sick more than a day or two or if you have questions about what to do.

EASY-TO-EAT FOODS FOR SICK DAYS

BREAD EXCHANGES	Amount (for 1 Exchange)	Approximate Calories
Bread: white, whole wheat	1 slice	70
white, whole wheat, toasted	1 slice	70
Cereal, hot	½ cup	70
Crackers		
Saltines	6 (2 inches square)	75
Soda crackers	4 (2½ inches square)	70
Graham crackers	2 (2½ inches square)	70

*The material in this chapter is adapted from *Diabetes Forecast*, May–June 1979.

BREAD EXCHANGES	Amount (for 1 Exchange)	Approximate Calories
Ice cream (vanilla, chocolate, strawberry)	½ cup (omit 2 Fat Exchanges)	170
Ice milk (vanilla, chocolate, strawberry)	½ cup (omit 1 Fat Exchange)	115
Jams or jellies, regular	1 level tablespoon	55
Jello, regular	⅓ cup	80
Popsicle*	½ twin pop	40
Pudding, plain (made with nonfat milk)	¼ cup	70
Sherbet	¼ cup	65
Soft drinks:		
Cola	4 ounces	55
Ginger ale	6 ounces	60
Soups, broth type	¾ cup	80
Soups, cream type (made with water)	1 cup (omit 1 Fat Exchange)	120
Sugar,* white granular	4 level teaspoons	60
Tapioca: whole milk, plain	⅓ cup	75

MEAT EXCHANGES	Amount (for 1 Exchange)	Approximate Calories
Cottage cheese (1–2% low-fat)	¼ cup	60
creamed	¼ cup (omit ½ Fat Exchange)	75
Custard, baked	½ cup (omit 1 Bread Exchange)	150
Egg substitute, low cholesterol	¼ cup	50
Egg, soft cooked or poached	1 (omit ½ Fat Exchange)	80
Eggnog,* commercial	½ cup (omit 1 Bread and 1 Fat Exchange)	170
Yogurt,* plain, skim milk	1 cup (omit 1 Bread Exchange)	120
Yogurt,* plain, whole milk	1 cup (omit 1 Bread and 1 Fat Exchange)	170

*Several foods have been included under more than one list to facilitate working them into your individualized meal plan.

VEGETABLE EXCHANGES	Amount (for 1 Exchange)	Approximate Calories
Tomato juice	½ cup	20
Vegetable cocktail	½ cup	25

MILK EXCHANGES	Amount (for 1 Exchange)	Approximate Calories
Eggnog* (nonalcoholic), commercial made with whole milk	½ cup (omit 2 Fat Exchanges)	170
Yogurt,* plain, skim milk	1 cup (omit 1 Fat Exchange)	120
Yogurt,* plain whole milk	1 cup (omit 2 Fat Exchanges)	170
Warm milk, skim	1 cup	80
Warm milk, low-fat	1 cup (omit 1 Fat Exchange)	125
Warm milk, whole milk	1 cup (omit 2 Fat Exchanges)	170

FRUIT EXCHANGES	Amount (for 1 Exchange)	Approximate Calories
Fruit juices, unsweetened		
Apricot, cherry, grapefruit, orange, peach	½ cup	40
Apple, pineapple	⅓ cup	40
Grape, prune, cranberry juice	¼ cup	40
Applesauce, unsweetened	½ cup	40
Applesauce, sweetened	⅛ cup (2 tablespoons)	30
Popsicle*	½ twin pop	40
Sugar,* granular	1 level tablespoon	45

Apricots, canned
   4 medium halves

---

*Several foods have been included under more than one list to facilitate working them into your individualized meal plan.

FAT EXCHANGES	Amount (for 1 Exchange)	Approximate Calories
Margarine	1 teaspoon	45

FREE FOODS	Amount (for 1 Exchange)	Approximate Calories
Fat-free broth, bouillon		
Coffee, regular or decaffeinated		
Tea		
Postum		

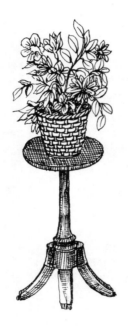

APPENDIX 1 □ Supplemental Exchange List

SUPPLEMENTARY VEGETABLE EXCHANGES

One Vegetable Exchange contains about 5 grams of carbohydrate, 2 grams of protein, and 25 calories. Each item listed is one Vegetable Exchange, using ½-cup serving unless otherwise noted.

Artichoke, globe (1 medium)
Bamboo shoots
Chinese vegetables
Green onions
Kohlrabi
Leeks
Mixed vegetables (⅓ cup)
Pea pods (snow peas)
Squash, summer (cocozelle, crookneck, scallop, spaghetti, straightneck, zucchini)

Tomato catsup (2 tablespoons)
Tomato paste (2 tablespoons)
Tomato puree (¼ cup)
Tomato sauce (not barbecue sauce)
Tomato, raw (1 medium)
Tomatoes, cherry (5–6)
Tomatoes, cooked or canned
Water chestnuts, canned (5–6 whole)

The following raw vegetables may be used as desired:

Celery cabbage
Chives
Coriander (cilantro)

Pimiento
Romaine

SUPPLEMENTARY FRUIT EXCHANGES

One Fruit Exchange contains 10 grams of carbohydrate and 40 calories. Each item listed may be used as one Fruit Exchange in the amount listed. The fruits listed are fresh, frozen, or canned without the addition of sugar.

Apricots, canned
  4 medium halves
Berries
  Boysenberries ½ cup
  Loganberries ½ cup
Cherries, red sour pitted ½ cup
Currants, dried 2 tablespoons
Figs, canned 1
Fruit cocktail, canned ½ cup
Grapefruit segments ½ cup
Grapes, Thompson's seedless
  ½ cup
Guava ½ medium
Kumquats 3
Lemon, whole 1
Limes 2
Melon, Casaba 1/10 melon or
  1 cup cubed

Melon balls or cubes 1 cup
Orange segments ½ cup
Peach, canned ½ cup or
  2 medium halves
Pear, canned ½ cup or 2 small
  halves
Pineapple, canned in pineapple
  juice 2 sliced drained or
  ½ cup chunks
Pineapple, crushed, canned in
  juice ⅓ cup
Pomegranate ⅓ medium
Raisins 1 small box (½ ounce)
Tangelo 1 medium
Watermelon 1 slice, approxi-
  mately 3 × 3 × 1 inch

SUPPLEMENTARY JUICE LIST

Apple cider ⅓ cup
Cranapple juice, low calorie
  1 cup
Cranberry juice, low calorie
  ¾ cup

Lemon juice ½ cup
Lime juice ½ cup
Orange-grapefruit juice ½ cup

SUPPLEMENTARY BREAD EXCHANGES

This list includes bread, cereal, and starchy vegetables. One Bread Exchange contains 15 grams of carbohydrates, 2 grams of protein, and 70 calories. Each item listed in the amount given may be substituted for one Bread Exchange. Note that some of the foods have added values from other Exchange Lists which must also be counted.

BREADS

Bread dressing ⅓ cup (omit 1 Fat Exchange)

Bread sticks 2 (9 inches long)

Croutons, plain 1 cup

French toast 1 slice (omit 1 Fat and 1 Meat Exchange)

Old world thin bread (flat bread, pita) 1 average

Party rye bread (small rounds) 4 slices

Taco shell 1 (6-inch diameter)

Very thin sliced bread 2 slices (approximately ¼ inch each)

CEREALS AND STARCHES

Barley, uncooked 1½ tablespoons

Cereals, concentrated bud types ¼ cup

Cereals, granola type ¼ cup (omit 1 Fat Exchange)

Cornstarch 2 tablespoons

Hominy, cooked ½ cup

Matzo meal 3 tablespoons

Oatmeal or rolled oats, dry ¼ cup

Tapioca, granulated 2 tablespoons

Wheat Germ ¼ cup

CRACKERS

Animal crackers 8

Cheese tidbits 30 (omit 1 Fat Exchange)

Melba toast 4 rectangles or 8 rounds

Pretzels approximately 70 thin 2¼-inch sticks

Rusk 2

Shredded wheat crackers 5 (omit 1 Fat Exchange)

Zwieback toast 3

SOUPS (Homemade or commercial, diluted with water according to label. Skim off visible fat.)

Broth-base: chicken noodle, chicken vegetable, beef noodle, vegetable beef 1 cup

Cream: celery, mushroom, tomato 1 cup (omit 1 Fat Exchange)

Pea-Bean: bean, chili bean, split pea ½ cup

STARCHY VEGETABLES

Corn, cob (5 inches long)   1
Corn, cream style   ¼ cup
Corn, whole kernel   ⅓ cup

Squash, winter (acorn, butternut, hubbard)   ½ cup

SUPPLEMENTARY MEAT EXCHANGES

Each item listed is one Meat Exchange if used in the amount indicated. Note that some of the foods have added values from other Exchange Lists which must also be counted.

LEAN MEAT EXCHANGES (7 grams of protein, 3 grams of fat, and 55 calories)

Cheeses: low-fat, containing 3 grams fat or less per ounce (read label)   1 ounce
Cholesterol-free egg substitute   ¼ cup
Dried beans, peas, lentils, chick peas (garbanzo), lima, navy, pinto, soy, split peas   scant ½ cup (omit 1 Bread Exchange)
Soybean curd (tofu)   3 ounces

MEDIUM-FAT MEAT EXCHANGES (7 grams of protein, 5 grams of fat, and 75 calories)

Beef, lean, ground   ¼ cup, cooked, drained

HIGH-FAT MEAT EXCHANGES (7 grams of protein, 8 grams of fat, and 100 calories)

Cheeses, natural: blue, brick, Camembert, Cheddar, Colby, Edam, Feta, Gouda, Limburger, Muenster, Provolone, Romano, Roquefort, Swiss   1 ounce
Cheeses, processed: American, pimiento, Swiss, cheese food, cheese spread   1 ounce
Cocktail frankfurters   3
Sausage links, brown-and-serve   2 (omit 1 Fat Exchange)
Vienna sausages   3 (omit ½ Fat Exchange)

SUPPLEMENTARY FAT EXCHANGES

One Fat Exchange contains 5 grams of fat and 45 calories. In the amount given, each item listed may be exchanged for one Fat Exchange. Foods that are primarily polyunsaturated fats are in capital letters.

Chicken fat   1 teaspoon
Chitterlings, fried   2 tablespoons
Coconut, fresh or processed, shredded or flaked   2 tablespoons
Cracklings   1 rounded teaspoon
Dressings (commercial):
   Cheese-flavored   2 teaspoons
   TARTAR SAUCE   2 teaspoons
   THOUSAND ISLAND (Low calorie)   2 tablespoons
MARGARINE, DIET (made with corn, cottonseed, safflower,
   soybean, or sunflower oil only)   2 teaspoons
MARGARINE, WHIPPED (see item above)   2 teaspoons
NUTS, CHOPPED   1 tablespoon
SEEDS
   PUMPKINSEED KERNELS   1 tablespoon
   SESAME SEEDS   1 tablespoon
   SUNFLOWER SEEDS, HULLED   1 tablespoon

SUPPLEMENTARY FREE FOODS

Note that the use of some of these foods should be limited as shown.

BEVERAGES
Broth or bouillon, fat-free
Carbonated beverages, sugar-free
Cereal beverages (1 cup per meal)
Clear consomme
Club soda, carbonated water (not tonic water or quinine water)

Cocoa, unsweetened (1 tablespoon per day)
Coffee lightener, liquid or powder (1 teaspoon per meal)
Soft drink mix, unsweetened powder

MISCELLANEOUS

Ascorbic acid powder (for canning and freezing fruits)
Bacon-flavored bits (1 teaspoon per day)
Baking powder, baking soda, cream of tartar
Chewing gum, sugar-free
Flavoring extracts
Gelatin, unflavored plain
Gelatin, flavored unsweetened (½ cup per meal)
Herbs, seasonings, spices
Jams and jellies, dietetic (1 teaspoon)
Meat sauces, commercial: catsup, soy, steak sauces (1 tablespoon
    per day)
Pancake syrup, dietetic (1 tablespoon)
Rennet tablets
Vegetable pan spray
Whipped topping, low calorie (1 tablespoon)
Yeast, baker's

SPECIAL OCCASION FOODS

These are regular sweetened foods, with the exception of the pudding, which may be used for special occasions—provided special occasions don't happen every day! For more frequent use ask your physican or diet counselor about how to include sugar-containing foods in your meal plan.

	Amount	*Exchange*
Cake, angel food (plain)	1½-inch cube (scant 1 ounce)	1 Bread
Cake, pound	1 ounce	1 Bread and 2 Fat
Cake, sponge	1½-inch cube	1 Bread
Chow mein noodles	½ cup	1 Bread and 1 Fat
Custard, baked	½ cup	1 Bread and 1 Fat
Doughnut, plain, cake type	1 small	1 Bread and 1 Fat
Gelatin, sweetened	½ cup	1 Bread
Ginger snaps	3	1 Bread and ½ Fat
Ice cream (vanilla, chocolate, strawberry)	½ cup	1 Bread and 2 Fat
Ice cream, soft serve	1 small cone	1 Bread and 1 Fat
Ice cream cone, waffle type (not sugar cone)	1	Free
Ice milk (vanilla, chocolate, strawberry)	½ cup	1 Bread and 1 Fat
Pudding (low calorie made with skim milk)	½ cup	1 Bread
Sherbet	¼ cup	1 Bread
Vanilla wafers	5	1 Bread, ½ Fat

APPENDIX 2 □ Nutrition and Physiology Glossary

ALCOHOL An ingredient in a variety of beverages, including beer, wine, liqueurs, cordials, and mixed or straight drinks. Pure alcohol itself yields about 7 calories per gram.

AMINO ACIDS Basic building blocks of protein. They contain the chemical elements carbon, hydrogen, oxygen, nitrogen, and other inorganic elements.

CALORIE A unit used to express heat or energy value of food. Calories come from carbohydrate, protein, fat, and alcohol. Also called "Kilocalorie."

CARBOHYDRATE One of the three major energy sources in foods. Carbohydrates are subdivided into three groups, *monosaccharides* (one sugar group per molecule), *dissaccharides* (two sugar groups per molecule), *polysaccharides* (many sugar groups per molecule).

"Simple sugars" also used to refer to monosaccharides.

"Starch" is one of the polysaccharides.

Carbohydrates yield about 4 caloires per gram.

CHOLESTEROL A fatlike substance present in blood, muscle, liver, brain, and all other tissues throughout the body of man and animals and therefore in foods of animal origin. Cholesterol is a key part of the fatty deposits in the arterial wall in atherosclerosis.

DIGESTION The breakdown of foods by chemical processes in the digestive tract to simpler substances in preparation for absorption so the body can use them.

DIURETICS A drug that stimulates increased water excretion.

ENRICHMENT The addition of one or more nutrients to foods made from refined grains in amounts approximately equivalent to those found in whole-grain products.

ENZYME A protein substance that speeds up chemical reactions but is not itself affected in the process.

FAT One of the three major energy sources in food. Fat yields about 9 calories per gram.

FIBER An indigestible part of fruits, vegetable, whole-grain cereals, and grains. Fiber is important in the diet as roughage, or bulk.

FOOD EXCHANGE Foods grouped together on a list according to similarities in food values. Measured amounts of foods within the group may be used as tradeoffs in planning meals. A single Exchange contains approximately equal amounts of calories, carbohydrates, proteins, and fats as other foods in the *same* list.

FORTIFICATION The addition of one or more nutrients to a food whether or not they are naturally present. The term "vitamin added" or "with added vitamin(s) and mineral(s)" as well as the term "fortified" have been used to identify fortified products.

HORMONE A chemical messenger. Hormones are secreted by a variety of glands in the body. Each hormone affects a specific tissue or organ and causes a specific response. Insulin is a hormone secreted by the pancreas.

POLYUNSATURATED FAT Fats from vegetable oils such as corn, cottonseed, sunflower, safflower, and soybean oil. Oils high in polyunsaturated fats tend to lower the level of cholesterol in the blood when used to replace part of the saturated fat.

PROTEIN One of the major nutrient groups in foods that are essential for the life processes. Proteins are made up of amino acids of which there are 22. Protein provides about 4 calories per gram.

SATURATED FAT   Fat that is often hard at room temperature, primarily from animal food products (like butter and meat fat). Examples of saturated vegetable fats are palm and coconut oil.

VITAMINS   Organic compounds which are found in small amounts in foods and are essential for many body processes; fat-soluble: A, D, E, and K; water-soluble: ascorbic acid and the B complex.

APPENDIX 3 □ Glossary of Cooking Terms

BAKE   To cook by dry heat in an oven; recipe may specify covered container.

BASTE   To moisten food during cooking to prevent dryness and add flavor. Unless otherwise stated in recipe, the juice or liquid in the pan is used for basting.

BEAT   To stir briskly by hand or with beater or electric mixer.

BLEND   To mix two or more ingredients together thoroughly.

BREAD   To coat with crumbs, or with a liquid mixture and then crumbs.

BROIL   To cook by direct heat.

CHILL   To cool thoroughly but not freeze.

CHOP   To cut into small pieces with knife, chopper, or scissors.

CUT IN   To combine fat with dry ingredients, using knives or a pastry blender.

DASH   Less than ⅛ teaspoon of an ingredient.

DICE   To cut food into small cubes, usually less than ½ inch square.

DUST   To coat lightly, as with flour.

DUTCH OVEN   A deep cooking utensil with tight-fitting cover.

FOLD   To combine ingredients with a gentle motion by cutting; to cut down through a mixture with a spoon or spatula and then bring it across the bottom of bowl and up side of bowl.

FRY   To cook in hot fat.

KNEAD   To use the hands to work dough on a floured surface to develop gluten.

MARINATE   To allow ingredients to stand in a liquid (usually mixture of oil with vinegar and lemon juice) to tenderize or enhance flavor.

MINCE   To chop finely.

RECONSTITUTE   To restore concentrated foods, such as frozen orange juice or dry milk powder, to their normal dilution by adding water according to package directions.

SAUTE   To cook in a small amount of fat.

SHRED   To cut or tear into small pieces.

SIMMER   To cook in a liquid over low heat just below boiling point.

TOSS   To mix ingredients lightly.

WHIP   To beat rapidly to incorporate air and increase volume.

SUGAR: WHAT'S IN A NAME

GLUCOSE   A monosaccharide (simple sugar) found in the blood, either derived from digested food or made by the body from other carbohydrates and from protein.

DEXTROSE   Another name for glucose.

FRUCTOSE   The sugar found in fruit, juices, and honey.

LACTOSE   The sugar found in milk.

MALTOSE   A sugar formed by the breakdown of starch.

SUCROSE   Table sugar.

GRANULATED SUGAR   Sucrose.

CONFECTIONER'S SUGAR   Powdery sucrose.

BROWN SUGAR   Sucrose crystals covered with a film of syrup.

CORN SUGAR   Sugar made from cornstarch.

CORN SWEETENER   A liquid sugar made from the breakdown of cornstarch.

CORN SYRUP   A syrup made by the partial breakdown of cornstarch.

HONEY   A syrup made up mostly of fructose.

INVERT SUGAR   A combination of sugars found in fruits.

MAPLE SYRUP   A syrup made from the sap of the sugar maple tree.

MOLASSES   Syrup that is separated from raw sugar during processing.

MANNITOL   A sugar alcohol that is broken down in the body the same way as other sugars but absorbed more slowly.

SORBITOL   A sugar alcohol produced by hydrogenation of glucose and invert sugar and absorbed more slowly than ordinary dietary sugar.

SORGHUM   Syrup made from sorghum grain.

APPENDIX 4 □

GUIDE FOR COMMON MEASUREMENTS

$$3 \text{ teaspoons} = 1 \text{ tablespoon}$$
$$16 \text{ tablespoons} = 1 \text{ cup}$$
$$8 \text{ fluid ounces} = 1 \text{ cup}$$
$$1 \text{ liquid pint} = 2 \text{ cups}$$
$$1 \text{ liquid quart} = 4 \text{ cups}$$
$$16 \text{ ounces} = 1 \text{ pound}$$

METRIC UNITS

Nutrition labels show the amounts of some nutrients in metric units rather than ounces. Here is a guide to help you read nutrition labels:

$$1 \text{ pound} = 454 \text{ grams (g)}$$
$$1 \text{ ounce} = 30 \text{ grams (g)}$$
$$1 \text{ gram} = 1000 \text{ milligrams (mg)}$$
$$1 \text{ milligram} = 1000 \text{ micrograms (mcg)}$$

ONE "CUPFUL"

$$\text{Granulated sugar} = 7 \text{ ounces}$$
$$\text{Butter} = \tfrac{1}{2} \text{ pound}$$
$$\text{Lard} = \tfrac{1}{2} \text{ pound}$$
$$\text{Flour} = 4\tfrac{1}{4} \text{ ounces}$$
$$\text{Rice} = 7 \text{ ounces}$$
$$\text{Cornmeal} = 5\tfrac{1}{4} \text{ ounces}$$
$$\text{Stale bread crumbs} = 1\tfrac{1}{2} \text{ ounces}$$
$$\text{Chopped meat, cooked} = 4\tfrac{1}{2} \text{ ounces}$$

APPENDIX 5 □
The U.S. RDA's and Your Diet

The U.S. RDA's (U.S. Recommended Daily Allowances) were set by the Food and Drug Administration for use in nutrition labeling and for labeling dietary supplements and special dietary foods. They are based on the National Academy of Sciences, National Research Councils' Recommended Daily Dietary Allowances. Generally, the highest value for each nutrient given in the NAS-NRC-RDA was adopted.*

Information on the vitamin and mineral content of foods is indicated on the lower part of the nutrition label. Listed are the percentages of the U.S. RDA's per serving for protein and at least 7 vitamins and minerals.

The label provides an easy way to compare foods to see which ones are better sources of certain vitamins, minerals, and protein. This information can help you select a more nutritious diet.

For your reference, the U.S. RDA's for adults and children 4 or more years of age are:

Protein   65 grams
Vitamin A   5000 International Units
Vitamin C (ascorbic acid)   60 milligrams
Thiamine (Vitamin B_1)   1.5 milligrams
Riboflavin (Vitamin B_2)   1.7 milligrams
Niacin   20 milligrams

---

*From HEW Publication No. (FDA) 77-2072, U.S. Department of Health, Education and Welfare, Public Health Service, Food and Drug Administration, 5600 Fishers Lane, Rockville, Maryland 20852.

Calcium   1.0 grams
Iron   18 milligrams
Vitamin D   400 International Units
Vitamin E   30 International Units
Vitamin B_6 2.0 milligrams
Folic acid (folacin)   0.4 milligrams
Vitamin B_{12} 6 micrograms
Phosphorus   1.0 gram
Iodine   150 micrograms
Magnesium   400 milligrams
Zinc   15 milligrams
Copper   2 milligrams
Biotin   0.3 milligrams
Pantothenic Acid   10 milligrams

APPENDIX 6 □ Selected Sources of Reliable Information

For additional information on Nutrition and Diabetes:

The American Diabetes Association local chapter.
The American Dietetic Association district chapter.
Call "Dial-a-Dietitian" in your local area.
Nutritionists—local Health Department.
Nutritionists—local county Agriculture Extension Service, U.S. Department of Agriculture.

INDEX □